Hypnosis for Spiritual Distress

This book synthesizes the work of Paul Tillich, Henry Nelson Wieman, and Joseph Murphy into an adaptable hypnotic protocol to be used with individuals experiencing spiritual distress. Spiritual distress is a nursing diagnosis of impaired ability to experience and integrate meaning and purpose in life through the individual's connectedness with self, others, art, music, literature, nature, or a power greater than oneself. This is often experienced as a result of a confrontation with mortality.

The central curriculum is supplemented by additional perspective on attachment theory, Buddhism, ethics, competencies, and spirituality.

The Clergy Special Interest Group
of the National Guild of Hypnotists
is a voluntary association of ordained and lay ministers,
professional and hobby hypnotists,
and others interested in
promoting and facilitating exploration and work
at the intersection of spirituality and hypnosis.
www.ngh-csig.net

Hypnosis for Spiritual Distress

Rev. Christian Skoorsmith, MA, PsyD(c), CI, FNGH (Editor)

originally
"Spiritual Hypnotism"
A Certification Curriculum of the National Guild of Hypnotists
written by
The Rev. Dr. C. Scot Giles, DNGH, OB
The Rev. Dr. Lindsay Bates, BCH, OB
on behalf of
The Clergy Special Interest Group
of the National Guild of Hypnotists
Original Copyright © 2007, National Guild of Hypnotists

Edited and expanded in 2024 by Christian Skoorsmith,
with supplemental material by Dr. C. Scot Giles, Celeste Hackett,
Dr. Timothy Jones, Dr. Carl G. Jung, Chris Lemig,
and Christian Skoorsmith.
Copyright © 2024 National Guild of Hypnotists

Published by
WholeHealth Publishing
Seattle, WA, USA
2024

First published 2024
by WholeHealth Publishing
9451 35th Ave SW, Seattle, WA 98126

WholeHealth Publishing is an imprint of WholeHealth Hypnosis

Typset in Cambria & Bahnschrift Light

Skoorsmith, Christian (Ed.)
Hypnosis for Spiritual Distress
(Includes bibliographical references and creative commons material.)
ISBN 978-1-304-27908-8 (paperback)

Hypnosis for Spiritual Distress

Rev. Christian Skoorsmith, MA, PsyD(c), CI, FNGH (Editor)

originally
Spiritual Hypnotism
**A Certification Curriculum of
the National Guild of Hypnotists**
written by
The Rev. Dr. C. Scot Giles, DNGH, OB
The Rev. Dr. Lindsay Bates, BCH, OB

Contents

Preface

by Christian Skoorsmith

"Spiritual Distress" is a term found predominantly in the nursing world and refers to a disturbance in a person's belief system, and the loss of those psycho-emotional resources, brought on by a confrontation with mortality or the reality of death. If profound enough, it can qualify as a diagnosis defined as "a disruption in the life principle that pervades a person's entire being and that integrates and transcends one's biological and psychological nature" (North American Nursing Diagnosis Association [NANDA], 1999, page 67). There is a deep need among this population for competent professionals to assist them in facing the manifold challenges of one's death becoming so stark a reality. As fewer hospitals employ full-time chaplains, and as American society grows less presumptively "Christian," trained and sensitive hypnotists can participate in the community of helping professionals attending to the subclinical/subdiagnostic dynamics of spiritual distress.

The core material in this book was developed more than seventeen years ago, as part of a training curriculum for people interested in using hypnosis in the course of spiritual work – primarily hypnotists who had seminary training and who served in some professional capacity an established religious community, but also hypnotists who served religious or spiritual clientele more generally. It was designed by two clergy hypnotists with extensive experience working with people dealing with cancer and facing terminal illness. They described the training as "Spiritual Hypnotism."

Quickly, however, a marketing problem arose centering around associations with the word 'spiritual.' Hypnotism is a professional community which is adjacent to and friendly with more metaphysical helping practitioners, so many attendees at these early trainings were expecting coverage of topics such as past-lives, spiritual warfare, energy-work, 'dark force' entities, Spirit Guides, Akashic records, and so on. Without implying any disparagement of those interests, it simply wasn't what *this* training was designed for, and those attendees were understandably disappointed. As a result, this curriculum was shelved for a number of years, and a tremendously valuable resource was effectively removed from the world of professional hypnotism.

In 2023, the Clergy Special Interest Group (CSIG) of the National Guild of Hypnotists pivoted direction. We decided to lean into our mission to "promote and facilitate exploration and work at the intersection of spirituality and hypnotism." An element of this was to open participation up to a broader scope of hypnotist and to actively encourage hypnotists and others to contribute to the study and application of hypnosis in spiritual pursuits. Integral to that vision is providing more responsible, ethical, and practical resources for addressing spiritual needs. This book is a first step in that direction, a resource that represents the particular strengths of rigorously trained and broadly experienced professional clergy.

The central content of this book is the product of Doctors Giles and Bates, seasoned professional ministers and trained hypnotists, bringing their years of education and pastoral experience to the task of formulating an introductory course on how to utilize hypnosis in a meaningful, ethical way within a spiritual-religious context. As the authors explain, this was developed with input from Christian and Jewish perspectives, and on the shoulders of two of the best theological minds of the twentieth-century. However, the central curriculum is not explicitly from one faith tradition. This book provides an orientation to broad human concerns that often find expression in spiritual language, ritual, and metaphor. Understanding these issues *as spiritual* brings perspective and resources to the work, regardless of one's religious orientation. Validating these concerns as legitimately spiritual – within a particular religious tradition or not – can itself be therapeutic. In this expanded edition, we welcome the experience and expertise of additional authors: some ordained, some uncredentialled but spiritually sensitive, and also outside the Judeo-Christian tradition.

While this curriculum was created by hypnotists with formal religious training and credentials, it was designed to be valuable for all hypnosis practitioners seeking to position themselves at the intersection of mind-science and spiritual concern. Overall, this book is focused on practicality and usefulness. While some helpful background is provided, the thrust of these pages is always directed at application in a therapeutic hypnotic context. As such, very few answers are provided here. This material teaches us how to meaningfully open doors, and how to help clients discover for themselves what is there for them – not to offer dogmatic principles, maps, or expectations. In this, the authors have been very brave as well as industrious. The brevity of this volume speaks to this point: this is a manual of practical tools for working with individuals to help them on their own spiritual journeys.

The structure of this book remains in most ways a curriculum best accompanied by a training. As such, it resembles notes rather than narrative, and is a skeleton or frame rather than a fully fleshed body. This is maintained as much as possible with an eye to efficiency: how best to convey information with the least interference. Again, the primary aim of this project is utility: what a hypnotist needs to know in order to get a good start doing this work. Of course, this is only an introduction to one variety of spiritually oriented hypnotism, and there remains much more to be explored.

Where helpful, I have added to the original 2007 curriculum for context or expanded on important, related topics, as well as updating some terms and topics that have changed since it was written. I have also supplemented the original curriculum with additional coverage of topics related to spiritual distress. While roughly a quarter of the material in the curriculum is my recent expansion, the bulk and essential organizing core remains the work done by Giles and Bates. The more obvious additions are the supplemental chapters on focused topics. These authors also begin to expand this resource beyond the narrow focus of terminal illness toward a general orientation around the faith dynamics of existential crisis.

I am grateful to Celeste Hackett for contributing a specialized form of parts work, included in the coverage of working with grief and loss. I am proud to welcome Chris Lemig's thoughts on how Buddhists wrestle with these issues and how hypnotists might meet their particular perspectives. Rev. Timothy Jones offers reflections on ethical concerns. I have also contributed two chapters: one using attachment as a lens for understanding religious experience, and another on ethical meaning-making in the face of suffering. Rev. C. Scot Giles graciously allowed inclusion of a recent keynote address he offered at the Heartland Hypnosis Conference on the topic of the spiritual core of hypnotism. This book also includes guidance by the American Counseling Association around competencies for this work, and an excerpt from a talk by Dr. Carl. G Jung to a group of Swiss Reformed clergy.

I extend my sincere appreciation to the Reverends Giles and Bates for their wisdom, effort, and integrity in bringing the core material together. The primary theological figures they invoke here, Henry Nelson Wieman and Paul Tillich, are among my favorite thinkers and bear worthy insights for everyone – clergy and lay, religious and secular. (An interesting historical note is that Rev. Dr. Martin Luther King, Jr.'s doctoral dissertation focused on Tillich and Wieman, together, as well. One can read that dissertation on Stanford University's MLK Institute website.) Giles and Bates' introduction of Dr. Murphy's work is a welcome application of suggestion in spiritual cause. I hope that in making this material more accessible as a stand-alone text, more people – in the NGH and the wider world – will find it as engaging and helpful as I do.

I also appreciate the permission of the National Guild of Hypnotists to update, edit, expand, and reprint this curriculum (as well as the generosity of Rev. Dr. Giles in providing the key text). The NGH remains the largest and oldest professional hypnosis organization in the world, and continues to serve as a 'big tent' under which many different voices and perspectives find mutual edification.

Hypnotism as a science, as a profession, and as a community continues to evolve. We hope bringing this valuable resource to light once again positively contributes to what we are becoming and what we bring to a world in need.

Christian Skoorsmith, Editor

2024 President,
National Guild of Hypnotists Clergy Special Interest Group

Introduction to the 2007 Curriculum
By C. Scot Giles & Lindsay Bates

In 1999 the National Association of Clergy Hypnotherapists, an independent organization of parish clergy, hospital chaplains and certified pastoral counselors merged with the National Guild of Hypnotists. To insure that the merged group would continue to meet the needs of its members, the merger agreement provided that membership in the new Clergy Special Interest Group (CSIG) would be limited to persons trained in accredited graduate theological schools who were or had been employed as clergy as their primary occupation.

This restriction was put in place so that the clergy members could continue to enjoy the fellowship of persons who shared similar training, and who could converse with each other about hypnotism from a perspective of ancient languages, systematic theology and a comprehensive background in Western church history. The CSIG was never intended to be a gathering of all clergy or spiritual persons, although it does aim to expand to include religious leaders in traditions other than Christian and Jewish. The CSIG is intended as a social and study group for those who share a common academic background. It bestows no credentials.

As time went on, the National Guild of Hypnotists asked the CSIG to create a curriculum on the spiritual use of the hypnotic arts and sciences. The requirements for this new certification curriculum were that the curriculum had to be broadly interfaith, and it had to hold up to academic analysis in terms of its subject matter and philosophy.

With this curriculum the CSIG presents the result of seven years of work. We have created a curriculum that we hope meets the request set before us.

Rather than favoring any particular faith tradition, we have gone to the work of three academic theologians, two of whom had distinguished careers as University-level faculty. Their names, Henry Nelson Wieman and

Paul Tillich, will be familiar to anyone who has studied theology at the collegiate level.

The third theologian, Joseph Murphy will be less well known to most. More of a popular figure during his lifetime than an academic theologian, Dr. Murphy did pioneer the interface between suggestion and religious practice in his writing, and seemed to us a good place to go for the practical techniques we included in this curriculum.

To provide a language for this curriculum we turned to the world of hospital chaplaincy. Chaplains work in a scientific environment where they are part of the health care team and function as interfaith providers of services. Therefore, the linguistic approach they favor seemed to us to be the best choice for speaking to the needs of many different persons with differing spiritual needs.

The CSIG has one regret in putting this material forward. While we had the benefit of Jewish, Catholic and Protestant clergy providing input to us as we created this material, we had no direct contacts with the Islamic, Buddhist or Hindu traditions available. We regret this, and hope someday to revise this material in light of the insights from those communities as well.

Section I:
Assessment, Profiling, and Goals

~ Working Definitions ~

Spiritual Hypnotism is the use of the hypnotic arts and sciences to help clients resolve issues of Spiritual Distress.

Spiritual Distress is the condition that develops when persons are unable to find meaning, love, inner strength and connection in their lives, or when there is conflict between what is happening in a person's life and what that person's beliefs state should be happening. Spiritual Distress can have a deleterious effect on mental and physical health.

A **Spiritual Hypnotism Provider** is a member in good standing of the National Guild of Hypnotists who has passed this certification curriculum and uses its methods with his or her clients. (Currently, this training is not actively being offered by the NGH. However, this language is preserved in this text as a recognition of past intent and of future hope.)

An **Instructor in Spiritual Hypnotism** is a Member in good standing of the Clergy Special Interest Group of the National Guild of Hypnotists who has taken and passed this curriculum as part of his or her continuing professional education.

(In 2024, the Clergy SIG added "Associate" status in order to open membership and participation to individuals interested in spirituality and hypnotism but had not received advanced degrees in religious training nor been professionally employed as an ordained minister. While Associates bring valued perspective to the group, this curriculum was designed with seminary graduates as instructors in mind. At present, however, since no training or certification is being offered, this point is moot.)

Spiritual Assessment is an appraisal of a client's presenting problem in terms of the sources of possible Spiritual Distress.

The **Spiritual Profile** is a summary statement of the Spiritual Assessment of the client expressed using a four-part acronym, HOPE.

The **Spiritual Goals Statement** is an expression of the changes a client might make, expressed using a four-part acronym, HOPE, that will result in the relief of the client's Spiritual Distress.

Spiritual Hypnotic Procedures are hypnotic methods conducted according to a five-step model that encourages a client to resolve his or her Spiritual Distress.

~ Technical Definitions ~

Spirituality is the human response to being alive and knowing that one has to die.

Almost everyone has a spirituality, although individuals may use different language to describe it, and it may or may not be a consistent match to that person's theology or religion. It is possible to have a spirituality without having a religion or a theology, but most spirituality is shaped, consciously or unconsciously, by the religious and theological positions and expressions of one's primary family and cultural groups.

Theology is a set of ordered propositions and definitions used to explain why the universe works as it does.

A theology does not require a belief in a deity. For example, Buddhist Theology is often atheistic.

Some people will have a very casual theology, while others will have studied it in a systematic way, and have a correspondingly greater awareness of how the definitions and propositions relate to each other.

One can have a theology without having a religion or a spirituality. For example, a person might endorse Superlapsarianism (the proposition that some institutions, such as marriage, existed before humanity fell from grace with God in Christian Theology) because he or she believes it is consistent with scriptural tradition without seeing that it could have any impact of his or her spirituality or faith tradition.

Religion is the cultural or social practice expressing the theology of a specific historical community.

One can have a religion without having a specific spirituality. However, one must possess a theology (however casual) to distinguish a religious or spiritual cultural or social practice from expressions of nationalism, popular culture or ethnic tradition. For example, Kwanzaa is a secular ethnic tradition that is not a religious practice, as it is not tied to a proposition about how the universe works.

~ Limits ~

Spiritual Hypnotism is not Metaphysical Hypnotism. Spiritual Hypnotism, as treated in and advanced by this curriculum, concerns itself only with the relief of Spiritual Distress. It does not concern itself directly with issues of reincarnation, spiritual possession or other supernatural or theological propositions.

The National Guild of Hypnotists has no theology. While the National Guild of Hypnotists believes that the hypnotic arts and sciences are useful tools in the hands of a properly trained practitioner to help persons resolve Spiritual Distress, the articulation of explicitly theological beliefs concerning afterlife, salvation, sin, theodicy, eschatology and other theological issues falls outside of the legitimate scope of the Guild.

Spiritual Hypnotism is holistic. In addition to hypnotism, a practitioner may recommend reading, meditation, prayer, social relationships or other lifestyle practices which complement and support the client's spiritual development.

So What Do I Do If....

Most healthy human beings live their lives within the context of a set of religious practices and spiritual beliefs. Becoming a Spiritual Hypnotism Provider does not mean you must lay your own personal spirituality, theology or religion aside.

When working with a client you should be clear about your own beliefs and practices if you think they might impact the welfare of your client. For example, if you believe a person is at fault or fundamentally unenlightened if they disagree with your specific spirituality, theology or religion, you might wish to restrict your Spiritual Hypnotism practice to those who share your fundamental views. Not doing so would likely produce a frustrating result for both you and your client.

Most Spiritual Hypnotism Providers, however, will 'bracket' their own spiritual, religious or theological beliefs when working with clients and make good faith efforts not to allow one's personal issues to affect the client encounter.

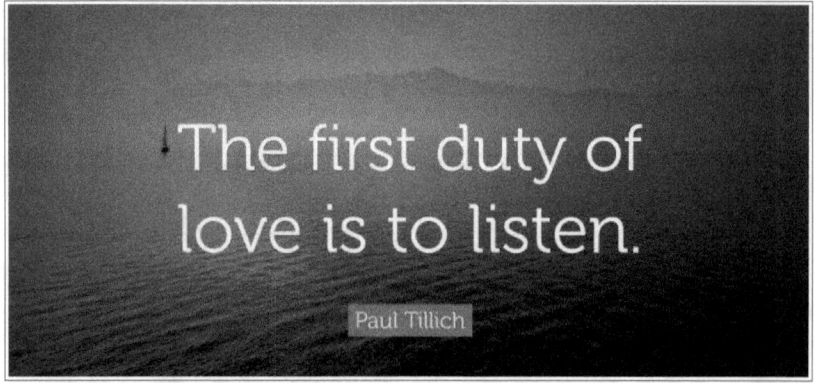

~ Spiritual Distress ~

The specific issues that might bring a client to seek out spiritual hypnotism will be as varied as the human species itself. Each person will have his or her own articulation of what is wrong.

Too often in the past Consulting Hypnotists have dealt with this by restating the client's issue in terms of the hypnotist's own theology, religion or spirituality. Then, the practitioner convinces the client that the client's problem is caused by something the hypnotist can respond to. After this, the hypnotist proceeds with some hypnotic procedure that has a spiritual tone. Examples might be past-life regression, spirit releasement, shamanic journeys, or other procedures specific to a particular theological, religious, or spiritual system.

In those cases where the client is suggestible and the hypnotist persuasive, this process might indeed work. However, it does violence to the integrity of the client who is encouraged (or coerced) to adopt a theological, religious or spiritual understanding that is not the client's own. Worse, this process will fail completely if the client is strong in their own understanding and refuses to adopt the prospective of the hypnotist.

To avoid this process we have created a new way of describing the client's issue: Spiritual Distress. To fill out this description, we turn to the work of theologian Paul Tillich (1886-1965), one of the foremost theologians of all time.

Tillich believed that human beings are unique in that we understand the meaning of time. Alone among living creatures, we understand that the world existed before we were born and will exist after our death. Other animals seem to show no such awareness.

The fact that we know we must die (and the world will persist) raises for us an issue about whether or not our life has any meaning. Are we here for a reason? If so, what is that reason? Spirituality and religion, as these authors understand it, evolve from our attempt to answer those two questions.

As we go through our lives and our understanding of the world changes, we give different answers to these two great questions. An answer that may have worked for a time will often be discovered lacking, and gets replaced with a better answer. For example, the child deals with the death of a neighbor by saying "only old people die because they've done what they were here to do," but has to replace this answer when a playmate dies in a sudden accident.

The difficulty all people have in answering this question gives rise to what Tillich called "angst," the German word for "fear." In English, the word angst connotes apprehension, insecurity, or anxiety. To avoid a confusion with the use of the word "anxiety" in modern psychology, and to specify the particular focus we are drawing from Tillich, in this process we use the phrase "Spiritual Distress."

Human beings strive to live meaningful lives; constantly striving to discover a pattern to events that gives meaning to our lives. When we are happy with the understanding we have about why the universe works as it does, we feel optimistic and purposeful. (This is true even of the most nihilistic philosophies, taking heart in a capacity to face the inanity of a meaningless universe with aplomb and courage, for instance. If a philosophy or theology does not offer hope of one kind or another, it will not endure.)

However, when the answers we have been giving ourselves do not work well because something calls them into question, we experience Spiritual Distress. Whatever we had been using to give ourselves hope no longer does so. We are no longer certain of the meaning of our life. This is an uncomfortable feeling that touches us deeply.

If we do not resolve this feeling by finding a new basis for meaning and hope, we may become emotionally disordered as well as spiritually anguished, and our physical health may suffer as well.

Therefore, a client comes for Spiritual Hypnotism when the client experiences Spiritual Distress for whatever reason. The task of Spiritual Hypnotism is to help the client resolve that distress in a way that is client-directed, respectful of the client, and adapting to and drawing on the client's spiritual resources and understanding.

The client will use the language of their own religion, theology, or spirituality to describe the sort of Spiritual Distress they are having. The common thread among all such descriptions will be that something has happened to upset the client's understanding of how the universe works. The client is no longer sure that the universe has meaning and is trying to find a way to believe that again.

Sidebar: What You Should Know About Tillich

Paul Johannes Tillich (1886-1965) was a German-born theologian who fled the rise of the Nazi movement in his home country and came to America in the late 1930s. He became a distinguished professor at Union Theological Seminary in New York and later at Harvard Divinity School and the Divinity School of the University of Chicago, where he taught until his death.

Between 1952 and 1954 Tillich delivered the *Gifford Lectures*, one of the most prestigious honors in the academic world. These lectures were collected into Tillich's influential three-volume Systematic Theology, which took the theological world by storm.

Tillich believed that much of the disconnection between religion and society resulted from a problem with language. Religion had not updated its vocabulary into words that were understood by modern men and women. Instead, the churches tried to teach society its specialized language (concepts like sin, grace, atonement, etc.) and largely failed.

Using the language of modern psychology, Tillich attempted to restate the classic issues of religion into the language of existentialist psychology. In this way, sensitive secular people could understand what the churches talked about. To do this Tillich took church language seriously, but not literally.

As an example, Tillich argued that humans are finite beings (that is, we have a limited life span) and finite beings cannot really be "caused" by another finite being. Somewhere, there had to be something that got the whole process started. Therefore, he concluded that we must be supported by something that is infinite.

However, Tillich argued that all ideas of God held by the human community were too limited to really designate an infinite being, or as he called it, the "God beyond the gods." Tillich thought that the best understanding of God was "Being Itself" or "the Ground of Being," which is a complicated idea that goes beyond the scope of this curriculum.

Tillich published many books and articles during his lifetime. Probably the best place to get a taste of his thinking is his popular book The Courage to Be. Another highly recommended work is the short book Dynamics of Faith which can be particularly useful for individuals interested in offering perspective to the Spiritually Distressed. Tillich emphasized the symbolic nature of religious language, arguing that literal interpretations fail to acknowledge that religious language and symbols point beyond themselves and are fundamentally unsettling, rather than definitive. For instance, his unusual conception of faith.

Tillich described faith as the state of *being ultimately concerned* with something that gives meaning and purpose to life. It drives actions, decisions, and ways of living, and transcends mere belief or intellectual assent. Faith involves the whole person – mind, body, and spirit. Tillich characterized faith as a verb rather than a noun, it is something we *do*: a courageous stance in the face of life's challenges, the courage to confront existential anxieties and uncertainties.

Thus, faith and doubt are not opposites nor mutually exclusive. Doubt is, in fact, an essential component of faith. Genuine faith involves risk and the courage to embrace uncertainty. The opposite of faith is not doubt but idolatry, where finite realities (such as success, nationalism, or even religious institutions) are elevated to "ultimate concern," distorting true faith.

Faith therefore is not static, something grasped or understood – rather faith grasps *us*, evolving through experiences and growth, reflecting the tension between the finite and the infinite, between what is and what we are called into being. Faith is seen as a transformative process, constantly evolving through personal experiences and existential questions. It is a journey rather than a destination, emphasizing ongoing engagement and growth.

It can be profoundly helpful to hold out this working understanding of faith – wherein fidelity to it is evidenced by one's willingness to struggle, to engage the tension, to live into the discomfort and crisis where "old beliefs" no longer adequately serve new experience or expanded perspective.

"One who is grasped by the One Thing That is Needed has the many things under their feet. They are concerned, but not ultimately, and when lost, they do not lose the one thing they need and that cannot be taken from them."

It can be an enormous support to know what is one's *ultimate* concern. There will still be challenges, struggles, trials, and strife, but one can weather those storms. When in spiritual distress, such a foundation to life has often been lost or lost sight of. Understanding the experience of doubt and loss compounding the instigating experience helps us appreciate the nature of spiritual distress and glimpse a vision for how to help with it.

~ Spiritual Assessment ~

A practitioner of Spiritual Hypnotism begins by conducting a Spiritual Assessment of a client. To do this you begin by asking the client what is wrong. Listening closely, you codify the client's problem statement into four areas. Taken together, these four areas of concern constitute the Spiritual Profile of the client.

The Spiritual Profile of the client at the time of Assessment is assumed to contain a dysfunction, problem or life crisis, for otherwise the client would not be seeking help.

You will also formulate a Spiritual Goals Statement for your client. This is the target you will help your client hit.

One way to think of the difference between a Spiritual Assessment, a Spiritual Profile and a Spiritual Goals Statement is to remember that the Spiritual Assessment is an activity on the part of the hypnotist. It is something that a Spiritual Hypnotism Provider does, the process that creates the Spiritual Profile and Spiritual Goals Statement.

The Spiritual Profile and the Spiritual Goals Statement are descriptions, usually written, of the problem statement of the client and goals for that client for purposes of Spiritual Hypnotism.

It is not possible for there ever to be a written Spiritual Assessment about a client, because Spiritual Assessment is an activity. Consulting hypnotists do not create, offer, or provide assessments unless one is licensed to do so (as a licensed psychologist, for instance). On the other hand, the Spiritual Profile of the client will often be a document, or something that could be expressed in a document. This is also true for the Spiritual Goals Statement.

> The courage to be is rooted in the God who appears when God has disappeared in the anxiety of doubt.
>
> Paul Tillich

Spiritual Profile

A Spiritual Profile is taken using the acronym HOPE:

> **H –** Sources of Hope/comfort/strength/etc.
>
> **O –** Organized Religion and Beliefs
>
> **P –** Personal Spiritual Practices
>
> **E –** Effects of Spirituality

For example, a female client seeks help, reporting constant worry about death and uncertainty about whether or not her life has any meaning.

A working assumption is made that there is something amiss in the client's spiritual profile that is causing her problem. The problem "Fear of death and concern about life meaning" is the Effect of her current spirituality. So the practitioner now works backward through the HOPE profile to discover what has gone wrong.

During a session's conversational interview, the client discloses that she has essentially no private spiritual practices other than occasional "Arrow Prayers" in moments of intense crisis. She is a lapsed church member who came from a denomination where sin, punishment and retribution are major themes. She currently has no church community, few social relationships and nothing she depends on for comfort except food.

In this case, her Spiritual Profile might be written as such:

> **H –** Comfort food
>
> **O –** Lapsed practice of retribution-heavy Christianity
>
> **P –** Occasional pleas to God in times of crisis
>
> **E –** Fear of death and concern about life's meaning.

Some version of the client's problem statement about his or her Spiritual Distress is always the last item (item E) on the Spiritual Profile. The other factors that contribute to the Spiritual Distress form the other items on the Profile. Any of these may, in other situations, be a complaint or concern relevant for hypnotic intervention in and of itself.

For example, in the case given, the client's eating behavior may profitably be the subject of a separate hypnotic intervention to control weight, or one's relationship with food, or associations of distraction or self-soothing with food. However, for the purposes of this curriculum we will stay focused on spiritual issues.

Spiritual Goals Statement

Having done the Spiritual Assessment and arrived at a good Spiritual Profile, the hypnotist is now is a position to help the client determine what changes need to be made to resolve the Spiritual Distress. This will be expressed as the Spiritual Goals Statement.

The Spiritual Goals Statement is also expressed using the HOPE acronym. One way of thinking about this is that the practitioner will help the client go from the client's dysfunctional Spiritual Profile to a functional one. To do this, the Spiritual Goals Statement forms a "target" for spiritual change that will help the client shift from a dysfunctional Spiritual Profile to a functional one.

In the case under consideration, the client's Spiritual Goals Statement might be something like this:

> **H:** Client needs encouragement to find some center for her life that is more appropriate than abuse of food. Perhaps weight management hypnotism might be helpful.

> **O:** Client needs encouragement to seek a faith community or group where personally relevant and hope-inspiring ministry is provided. A referral to appropriate clergy may be helpful.

> **P:** Client needs encouragement to develop regular spiritual practice such as "Daily Walk Prayers," Mindfulness or Inspirational Reading. Helpful books or tapes might be recommended.

E: Client would be expected to lower her fear of death and to discover a meaning for her life. Personal journaling for self-monitoring,
and revisiting the concern on a SUDS scale with the hypnotist could
be helpful to gauge progress.

In all cases, the last item (item E) becomes an expression of what
would happen when the client's Spiritual Distress is resolved by Spiritual
Hypnotism. Ideally, some check-in measure or opportunity is built into the
client work (minimally at the beginning and again at the end) to monitor the
effectiveness of the intervention. Reassessing and drafting a revised Spiritual Profile (HOPE) could serve as a concluding document that the client
could turn to for grounding as they continue on their spiritual journey.

For the imaginary client in this example, she would find herself with
something healthy at the center of her life – a relationship, hobby, or ambi-
tion, perhaps. Having this need met in healthier ways, she would not be
turning to food for distraction or comfort and would be managing her
weight better. She would have a religious community where she felt welcome and a spiritual practice that is more comprehensive and stabilizing
than what she had before.

Therefore, after she has consulted a Spiritual Hypnotism Practitioner, this client might end up with a Spiritual Profile that looked something like this:

H: Client finds herself very involved with issues of deep ecology and
wholesome living. She feels a mystical connection to the earth.

O: Client participates in on-line discussion groups on environmental
awareness and has a circle of friends drawn from that community.
She meets quarterly with a group of people loosely connected to the
Wicca faith.

P: Client engages in personal rituals of earth-centered worship; including shamanic drumming, trance spirituality and maintains a
scratch organic kitchen as a spiritual discipline.

E: Client has a healthy natural lifestyle and feels herself deeply connected to the environment and natural world. She believes she will

be reincarnated somehow in the natural world after her death and feels this to be comforting.

Or, depending on what the client believes, it could look like this:

H: Client believes that the natural world is a creation of God and is full of the spiritual energy of Jesus.

O: Client is a member of the Four Square Gospel Fellowship and finds special enjoyment in its positive and motivational interpretation of scripture.

P: Client practices daily prayer and Bible reading. She maintains a trim weight by participating in a Christian weight management program that encourages members to feel their bodies must be kept as a fit temple for God.

E: Client believes that at death she will "be with" Jesus in some way and finds this a positive image.

The key thing to note is that the hypnotist does not determine how the client will fulfill the Spiritual Goals Statement and move toward a more functional Spiritual Profile. The client does that. The hypnotist simply serves as a guide enabling the client to fulfill whatever spiritual destiny the client has.

How you do this for a client comes later in this curriculum. For now, master the craft of Spiritual Assessment.

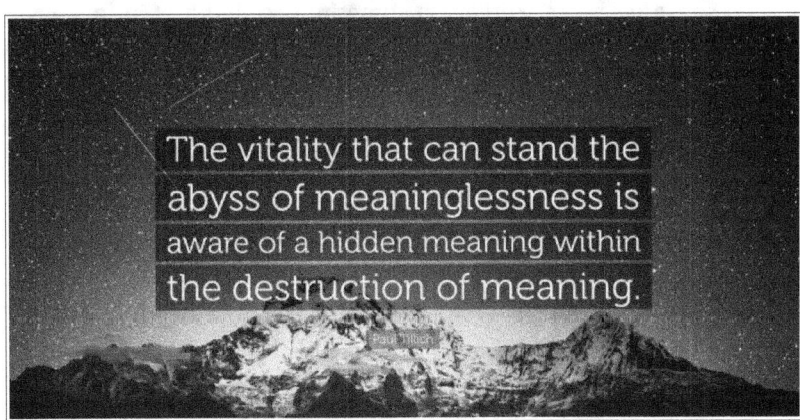

The vitality that can stand the abyss of meaninglessness is aware of a hidden meaning within the destruction of meaning.

Even Hovering Attention & Potential Space

It is of utmost importance to meet clients in spiritual distress with empathy, without judgmentalism, and with 'even hovering attention' to the diverse aspects of their experiences.

Some clients' previous experience with religion, spirituality, or spiritual 'leaders' may have been decidedly bad: hurtful, harmful, deceitful, full of hatred or judgment or mistreatment. The understanding and open context of hypnosis can provide a safe harbor, a corrective space in which acceptance, care, and empowerment can replace hateful rejection (by others or even themselves). This is a necessary starting point – but is often not where the 'gold' is to be found.

People are complex beings, of course, and our development is not always 'even' - we have blind spots, inner conflicts, defense mechanisms, strengths we built over time to compensate for weakness we may not be able to acknowledge. When we are focused exclusively on 'acceptance' and 'affirmation' we may inadvertently miss opportunities for the client to understand important (if uncomfortable) aspects of their own experience. At worst, we may unconsciously collude with the client's unconscious defenses against 'upsetting the apple cart,' missing a potentially productive insight or conversation.

We should engage clients without judgmentalism regarding their choices, but this should not therefore be a stance of unquestioning and final approval. When holding 'evenly hovering attention' we listen with both empathy and a detached observation, not assuming that what the client is consciously articulating is the whole story. It may not reflect everything they think or feel, or even be an accurate representation of the 'whole' of their experience. As more-or-less neutral parties, we can listen to our clients, suspending what they may have communicated or what we know of the 'facts' in order to understand the varieties of the client's experience and also allow space for other possibilities or perspectives to rise.

This sense of 'room to play' is sometimes called 'potential space' and points to a sense of freedom and possibility by the client. Given room to imagine, to engage what might feel unfamiliar, fraught, or on the edge of personal possibility is a priceless value. In our consultation, conversation, and hypnotic work, we should strive to cultivate for our clients a sense of permission to consider new dynamics, relationships, or possibilities – so unconscious material is more likely to rise into consciousness and also so that clients feel free to express new or alternative positions, attitudes, beliefs, or identities without judgment or pressure or permanence.

Rarely do any of us experience such acceptance and creative freedom. This is often even more true for people who may have in the past not felt welcome to process spiritual distress in a supportive community.

Section II:
The Spiritual Hypnotic Process

Once you have formed the Spiritual Goals Statement you are ready to design the hypnotic approach you will take to help your client move to a more functional Spiritual Profile.

While there are many ways one can do this, the clergy who designed this curriculum have created, tested and recommend a five-part method grounded in the work of another famous theologian, Henry Nelson Wieman.

While a person can, theoretically, design their own hypnotic process for spiritual purposes, such a process carries with it no authority. By grounding your hypnotic process in the thought of a great modern theologian you receive the benefit of working with ideas that have been checked out by other people over a long period of time and found solid. This is not dogma, but rather earnest insight provided by practitioners who have been held accountable by boards, deans, and religious communities, and the rich distillation of one of the world's most daring thinkers.

This five-part technique is drawn from the 1929 volume <u>Methods of Private Religious Living</u> by Henry Nelson Wieman. Dr. Wieman was one of the most respected theologians of his time and comes from the "Process Philosophy" movement along with Professors Alfred Whitehead, Charles Hartshorne, Henri Bergson, and John Dewey.

First, you hypnotize the client using any appropriate technique. Then, you deepen the client's trance using imagery and patter arranged in specific layers:

- **Part One:** The hypnotism opens with materials selected to remind the client of the Beauty and Mystery of our world and lives.

- **Part Two:** The hypnotic patter shifts to suggestions about the good that might be manifest in the life of the client because of that Beauty and Mystery.

- **Part Three:** The client is guided to reflect upon those issues with which the client struggles. This might be done in silence.

- **Part Four:** The client is guided to consider how his or her personal attitude might be re-adjusted to the purpose of living more successfully. This might be done using future pacing.

Then, you move to **Part Five**, which is called "The Master's Voice."

The Master's Voice

"The Master's Voice" is an appropriately authoritative, directive suggestion technique for Spiritual Hypnotism. Basically, you create a kind of affirmation for your client in Part Five. When you present to the client an affirmation that captures the change the client should make, you present this affirmation using "you" language so that the client hears the affirmation as if it were the statement from an external authority.

Clients are instructed to install a daily "quiet time" into their lives of 15-30 minutes. The quiet time can be at the beginning or end of the day. During the quiet time the client is instructed to work through the five steps of the method on his or her own: (1) reflection on beauty and mystery, (2) reflection on the possibilities for good, (3) reflection on one's personal struggles, (4) consideration of possible personal readjustments, and (5) interior voicing of the auto-suggestion using the imagined voice of the hypnotist or another familiar, spiritually-significant figure.

It is crucial to this method that the affirmation, even if it comes directly from the words of the client, be presented as if it were a pronouncement of truth and expectation by an external authority. For example, the hypnotist might say to the client, "You are happy with the body you have been given." During the quiet time the client imagines the voice of the hypnotist saying "You are happy with the body you have been given." The client does <u>not</u> say "I am happy with the body I have been given."

The reason for this approach is that in spiritual matters the mind often regresses to a childlike state where it internalizes any voice of authority. (Why this happens can be found addressed in the section "Attachment and Spirituality" below.) The goal of the suggestion is to make the subconscious mind of the client pregnant with the expectation of helpful change. Speaking as an external authority will do that in a way that by-passes the censor of the conscious mind that might disagree with the auto-suggestion if it were presented with "I" language.

For example, if one were to ask the client to say "I am happy with the body I have been given," the conscious mind of the client might easily respond with "the heck I am." Absent the authority of the Master's Voice, the client might inadvertently reinforce the negative refusal rather than the positive proposition.

However, if the suggestion is delivered to the hypnotized client by an external voice in a setting that feels authoritative, reverent and positive, the conscious mind is much more likely to respond with "yes, sir," or "yes, ma'am."

To use this technique effectively the hypnotist needs to have done their own inner work and resolved any authority issues that might prevent him or her from being directive in this way. Spirituality involves direction. Within the institutional church, the professionals who guide the spiritual formation of candidates for ordination are called Spiritual Directors for exactly this reason.

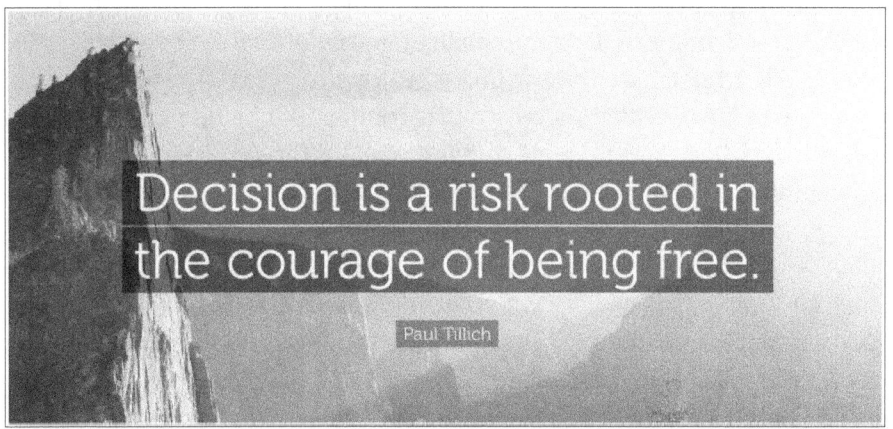

Decision is a risk rooted in the courage of being free.

Paul Tillich

Sidebar: What You Should Know About Wieman

Henry Nelson Wieman (1884-1975) was an American theologian who sought to unite religion and science. He enjoyed the support of many of the scientists of his day and that fame led to his appointment to the Divinity School of the University of Chicago in the 1920s. He would also hold distinguished teaching positions at several other universities during his lifetime.

Wieman belonged to an intellectual movement called Process Philosophy or Process Theology. That is, he believed that the fundamental nature of reality was an ever-changing process. In this process, one thing constantly transforms into something else. What prevents a universe of ever-transforming events from being simple chaos is that the process of transformation is guided by God, and God apparently seeks to move this process in certain directions.

What Wieman meant by "God" was also in process. Two of his most influential and accessible works are <u>The Source of Human Good</u> and <u>Man's Ultimate Commitment</u>, wherein he describes God as Creative Good as opposed to any created goods (in other words, "things"). God is creativity and a lure to deeper and richer experience.

However, God is not able to tell the future. While God knows all things, the future has not yet happened and therefore cannot be known. No one, including God, can know something that has not yet occurred. The future is probability and possibility, not fact. Only facts can be known. God can hope, encourage, and hold out possibility but cannot coerce or force.

What this means is that God is waiting to see what will happen to the universe God created (is creating, is coming into being in mutual relationship). As God tries to move things along, God has to contend with the momentum and influences created by what has already happened, and with what human beings are up to. God may be trying to make the Earth a paradise, but that would not stop human beings from blowing it up. The challenge for humanity is to work with God, not against God; to cultivate created good and not lose sight of Creative Good; to lean into greater possibility and richness of experience, even while knowing that it opens us up to experiencing more vulnerability and suffering, too.

The contribution Process Philosophy has made to modern thought has been enormous, and the Process Philosophers have had an impact on theology, mathematics, and physics. (Indeed, several of them have been primarily mathematicians or physicists.)

Wieman argued that to grasp what a person really believed, one had to discover what that person regarded as of "ultimate concern." Whatever in that person's belief system was taken with absolute seriousness was the "religion" for that person. Sometimes the abstract and heavily symbolized language of religious institutions is helpful for growing a sense of awareness in us what might be of ultimate concern. Sometimes, however, that language confuses or distracts us, too.

Traditional religious language describing "God" often gives primacy to the subject of the sentence ("God"), rather than the predicate (e.g., "is love"), placing our ultimate allegiance on the subject. Wieman was among thinkers who advocated switching the category to identify more clearly what one is worshiping – lean on the predicate: If God is love, then whatever is ultimately worthy of love is "God." If God is life, then what life is, is God; where we find life, we are finding God. Asking ourselves what our predicate clauses about God are (how we describe who or what God is) more directly indicates to us what our ultimate concern really ought to be.

Some people have understandings of religion that are universal and just. Others have understandings that are much more limited (such as believing that only the members of one church community are good) while others, even if they denied it, really worship things which were more like "idols." For example, Wieman believed that some people really had money or power as their religion, even if they dressed that up in other words.

In Wieman's view, a constant temptation for humanity is the over-identification with and worship of creat*ed* goods, things we can hold, handle, or wrap our heads around. One devotional aim he had was to reorient humanity: while we enjoy and value created goods, our ultimate loyalty is beyond our own provincial priorities or viewpoints and to Creative Good. We can recognize the contingency of provisional values, perpetually holding out a daring loyalty to what might yet be discovered by/through/in an *ultimate* concern.

It is interesting to note that the above represents a similarity between Tillich and Wicman. Tillich believed "that at which we cannot laugh is the god of our idolatry – a mischosen ultimate concern."

At least two important principles should be articulated for our work with clients experiencing Spiritual Distress. First, much misunderstanding and suffering comes from our misplaced loyalties toward created things (even "good" things) and not holding our ultimate loyalty to the possibility of growth and new understanding (Creative Good – not a *thing* but a value that points beyond itself). Where we place our *ultimate* concern (alongside our provisional concerns, some of which are also important and worthy of attention and care) is our "real" religion.

Second, God cannot coerce; God can only Call. This is true for individual humans and also cancer cells and bomb fuses and distracted drivers and atmospheric rivers. The universe is not a puppet on a string for God to prance around. God wants the best for all of us and also recognizes the risk: greater capacity for joy, love, and experience also means greater capacity for brokenhearted-ness and suffering. It doesn't always work out, but how daring is a God that thinks the risk is worth it? We grow to feel *more* – an adventurous Something knows richer and deeper experience is so good, it is worth the risk. That tells us something about love, as well as life.

> Religion is the state of being grasped by an ultimate concern, a concern which qualifies all other concerns as preliminary and which itself contains the answer to the question of a meaning of our life.
>
> Paul Tillich

~ Practical Wisdom from Wieman ~

Henry Nelson Wieman's philosophy and theology can provide several streams of potential support for someone experiencing spiritual distress. When working with a client, of course, it is not necessary (or advisable) to provide a lesson on the philosophy of Wieman (or anyone else). Understanding Wieman in the following ways helps *us* by holding out different, deeper, potentially transformative reframes of our experience (and that of our clients). Importantly, both Tillich and Wieman did not avoid troubling questions or the discomfort of having one's core convictions shaken (even crumbled). They did not offer Pollyanish platitudes that dismiss the reality of the suffering caused by those experiences. Their understandings of the human struggle put those experiences and the growth that comes from them at the center of human life.

Our clients who have come to us in spiritual distress are struggling with *Meaning*, with a capital 'M.' While it is not often helpful in the darkest moments to cast it so, we can hold that sense in our hearts and minds as we companion them in this process. Tillich and Wieman help us keep this growth-oriented understanding of Meaning at the forefront of our thoughts and work, so we can embody that perspective for our clients to absorb implicitly and, eventually, explicitly.

Three key takeaways from Wieman might serve us well in our work with those in spiritual distress.

First, **a focus on human good**. Wieman emphasizes identifying and fostering the sources of human good. This might seem counter-intuitive, given Wieman's focus on the creative good of the Divine. However, good in this world *is* good! God, in Wieman's view, wants us to experience good more deeply, richly, and consistently! (God, Spirit, Creative Good, the Universe, Source, Ahura Mazda – however one conceives this – wants so much for us to experience good richly, that it is worth the risk of us feeling pain to that same extent.) So, by focusing on what brings genuine value and meaning to life, individuals can find a constructive path forward even amid distress. This perspective shifts attention from abstract theological debates to concrete actions that enhance well-being and community.

Wieman advocates for an understanding of God based on human experiences of goodness and creativity rather than speculative metaphysics. This can be comforting for those struggling with doubt, as it grounds spirituality in tangible experiences of love, justice, and beauty, making the divine more accessible and relatable.

Second, Wieman casts **Creative Process as (the) Divine**. Growth is great, of course, but *experience* itself (Tillich calls it Being) is our participation in the divine process/personality. Even struggling. Wieman's view that God is the creative process at work in the world is an opportunity individuals see their struggles and growth as part of a divine process. Pain or feeling stuck, lost, abandoned, hopeless... that is *being*, too. They are an experience of the holy, as well. Understanding our struggles in this way can reconnect us with our source of meaning, or at least hold out hope of reconnection (recognizing our "connection" was never really lost). Recognizing that creativity and transformation are inherently valuable can inspire hope and resilience in times of hardship.

By emphasizing the intrinsic value of rich and meaningful experiences, Wieman's philosophy encourages individuals to seek out and appreciate the depth of their lived experiences. This can help individuals in spiritual distress find purpose and joy in everyday life, even amid suffering.

Finally, Wieman suggests that faith is more about the functional role of divine good in our lives rather than rigid doctrines. What that means for us is that **specific "beliefs" or tenets or doctrines are not Faith**. Sometimes spiritual distress is experienced because of (or in the midst of) some tenet or particular belief no longer feeling true – and having been told that belief *in that teaching* was what faith is, feeling a loss of faith (or goodness, or qualification, or worthiness, or sense). Really grasping that faith is not evidenced by or experienced in particular ideas/beliefs/tenets, but rather is the leaning-in to life and openness to the insights that rise from experience, can shift one's experience of loss. No longer is the Holy withdrawn. In fact, if anything, the disruption of what was held dear has brought it nearer. This approach allows for a flexible and personalized spirituality that can adapt to individual needs and circumstances, providing a more inclusive and supportive framework for those in distress.

Instead of being torn away from the Divine, Wieman helps us see our experiences – even the painful and disruptive ones – as creativity unfolding, or at least that bud of new growth being held out for us. This is not to "sugar-coat" or deny the reality of suffering – in fact, quite the opposite. To the extent that we are *really* open to joy and love, we may experience that degree of suffering and loss. But, like an adventurous God, we can lean into rather than away from our experience, if we see the risk as worth it.

Creating the Auto-Suggestion

The first four parts of the Spiritual Hypnotic Process are intended to align the client's mind with all that is good and true in the universe, as that is understood by the client. Another way to think of this is that these steps encourage the client to adopt a hopeful positive mental attitude about spiritual things.

Your success or failure in doing Spiritual Hypnotism rests on your skill in facilitating the final step, the creation of the Auto-Suggestion that will move the client in the direction of the changes indicated by the Spiritual Goals Statement.

- Auto-suggestions are **simple declarative sentences**, using as few words as possible, that state what is desired as if it has already happened. These are sometimes called Affirmations.
- Auto-suggestions should **avoid negative words** and "painted" words that carry a strong negative emotional charge. For example, "cancer," "hate," "pain," and "lust" are painted words.
- Auto-suggestions must be **at least half believable**.
- The client repeats the auto-suggestion to themselves as if the hypnotist were saying the words. Therefore, the suggestions are constructed using **"You" rather than "I" language** and delivered using the Master's Voice.

In a sense, religion is a story. Every religion contains at its core the story of its creation, often organized around an account of the religion's founder. Stories provide a convenient way for a writer to convey a sense of meaning as a story contains a "plot" or a set of "themes" that hold the parts together.

As you create the auto-suggestion for your client you are helping the client change their personal story from one where the client is the Victim to one where the client plays the role of Victor. Some teachers of theology argue that this change is at the core of all religious story.

The clergy who created this curriculum urge you to keep the following propositions in mind as you work with your clients. These propositions are drawn from the hypnotic theology of Joseph Murphy who pioneered the use of hypnotism in spiritual practice until his death in 1981.

Proposition #1: The Subconscious Mind is immensely powerful and can influence events. Miracles are possible. However, to use this power safely the mind must be attuned by certain principles. Attempting to use this power without such attunement results in personal disaster.

What you state in the auto-suggestion needs to conform in some reasonable way to the great teachings of the world's religious leaders as you understand them. For example, an auto-suggestion that expresses harm to another person is inappropriate.

Proposition #2: Belief is the connection between the Power of the Subconscious or Unconscious Mind and the Technique used to activate that power. That is, what allows a person to use Subconscious Power is that person's belief that the power can be utilized.

The auto-suggestion must conform to what the client believes, not necessarily what the hypnotist would personally agree with. For example, an auto-suggestion that expresses the hypnotist's belief in reincarnation or angels would be inappropriate if the client does not share that belief. On the other hand, if the client holds a belief in angel-guides but the hypnotist does not, it would be appropriate to craft an autosuggestion including such a belief – for it is the belief's power for the client, not for the hypnotist, that gives the suggestion its authority.

Proposition #3: Auto-Suggestion is a fact of life and goes on all the time. It can be Positive (which corresponds to religious principles) or Negative (which does not correspond to the teachings of the great religious leaders). Most personal difficulties are caused by Negative Auto-Suggestion, either caused by oneself (mistaken beliefs) or given by others (negative persuasion).

It is always appropriate to use protective and positive language in the auto-suggestion. For example, including words like "God watches over you" would likely be appropriate for most clients.

Proposition #4: Regular use of this technique establishes a connection between one's mind and something greater. This connection becomes stronger with practice and causes positive things to be attracted into the life of a person with such a connection. The religious name for this is *charisma*.

Do not be surprised if Spiritual Hypnotism sets off a positive chain of events in the life of your client. It is even reasonable for you to expect this.

Proposition #5: There is nothing wrong with Abundance nor with working with a client to attract Abundance.

Wealth is not un-spiritual and there is nothing wrong with working with a client so that he or she comes to believe he or she is worthy of abundance. The Golden Rule isn't just an ideal ethical principle, it's a fact of life. Most people do treat others as badly as they treat themselves, and that is why they are often unhappy and poor. The scriptural admonition to love our neighbors as we love ourselves is one of many religious expressions of that deep truth. Healthy love of self as a child of God (one possible phrasing) leads to acting lovingly toward others as well. And it should be no surprise that those who act lovingly, generously and kindly attract abundance in many forms into their lives.

Proposition #6: Beware Idolatry. Idolatry is defined as *"giving attention to or uniting with that which is negative and destructive."(Joseph Murphy, The Power of Your Subconscious Mind, p. 180)*

This is a generally more approachable definition of idolatry for most people than the potentially abstract and unusual (though powerful and profound) descriptions of Tillich and Wieman, but the three are related and mutually informative. For Tillich, idolatry is giving ultimate commitment to something that does not deserve it (often exemplified by any number of finite things that demand ultimate loyalty: organizations, nations, doctrines, parties, and so on). Wieman, for whom God was the Creative Good that transforms people as they could not transform themselves, idolatry was reducing God to an object in the material world or any concrete/static thing. The overlap among the three is the destructiveness of giving one's ultimate commitment (attention/focus/loyalty) to some*thing* that limits or takes away from the creative growth and transformation of the individual.

Murphy's description is more concrete and emotionally evocative, as it would need to be for a popular preacher of self-help. As such, it is easy to grasp, especially in times of crisis. According to Murphy, the best way to live is to unite with what is positive and life-affirming. Nagging another person is idolatry, as is abuse, resentment or ill will.

Sidebar: What You Should Know About Joseph Murphy

The Rev. Dr. Joseph Murphy (1898 – 1981) was the Minister Director of the Church of Divine Science in Los Angeles for 28 years. A hugely popular clergyman in his day, it is reliably reported that the average attendance at his worship services was 1300-1500 persons. His was one of the largest congregations in the world associated with the New Thought movement that, among other things, emphasized the mental aspect of sickness and the healing power of "right thinking." He retired from his pulpit in 1976 but continued to give popular radio addresses. He died at the age of 83.

His best-known book is <u>The Power of Your Subconscious Mind</u> (first published in 1963) which sold millions of copies. Throughout his career he routinely drew upon the hypnotic/mesmerist tradition by references to Emile Coue', Hippolyte Burnheim, Phinneas Quimby, and others. Similar to other works of the age (e.g., Think and Grow Rich), Murphy's book mixes popular psychology, individual empowerment, a loose interpretation of Christian theology, and American idealism in the ability to create a future of health and financial abundance for oneself, to create an inspiring step-by-step process that centers on consistently positive thinking, attitude, and disposition.

While not an academic theologian, and the nature of his hypnotic training is not documented, Dr. Murphy was indisputably the forerunner in the use of hypnotism in spirituality. His use of hypnosis was eminently practical, meant to be used by and for "the common man." No curriculum on this subject would be complete without some reference to him.

Process Theology

Several times in this curriculum, process philosophy is mentioned as one element in the background of this material. While this curriculum is not a product of process thought, process thought was part of the formative structure that enriches the tools and approach we introduce here. It is not necessary to be a process thinker, by any means, in order to utilize this material and be a spiritual hypnotism provider. However, more familiarity with process thought might further contextualize and enrich your use of these tools in this spiritual endeavor.

Process theology is a school of theological reflection that views reality as dynamic and evolving, emphasizing that everything is in a constant state of becoming rather than being static. Rooted in the process philosophy and metaphysics of Alfred North Whitehead, process theologians understand God as not an unchanging, omnipotent being but rather a participant in the ongoing process of the universe. This yields some unconventional but therapeutically fruitful implications about the universe, divinity, and humanity.

First is the sense of a profoundly relational God. Remember, "God," for process thinkers, is not a thing or even person or personality. Language is limited because we instinctively anthropomorphize the subjects of sentences. God is deeply involved in the world, influencing and being influenced by events. God is participatory to an extent that is unpalatable to Christian doctrines of an unchanging god who is removed from this world. In process thought, God is also growing (through/in/with us and all that is). This relational aspect means that God's knowledge and nature evolve with the unfolding of the universe.

This relational nature is not limited to "God" – especially as God is not a separate Other from the active emergence of Being. All of reality is seen as a series of interconnected events rather than static substances. Everything is in process, constantly changing and developing.

Genuine growth and change relies on actual freedom – which in process philosophy is a quality that pervades existence, if even in very small ways among smaller things (the cells in a carrot, for instance, have a narrower range of options from which to freely choose). In the complex combination of factors that make up a human being, the possibility of choice is much more rich. Though, as hypnotists, we recognize the powerfully shaping/directing influence of the subconscious mind, we nonetheless also land on the personal power and awareness of freedom. Similarly, process theology highlights the importance of human free will. God does not unilaterally control the world but works persuasively rather than coercively, allowing for genuine human freedom and creativity.

So, humans are co-creators with God, contributing to the ongoing creation and improvement of the world. This collaborative view encourages active participation in addressing social and ecological issues. However, humans are also free to make other choices, ones that lead to suffering. Process theology offers a nuanced understanding of evil and suffering, viewing them as inherent aspects of a dynamic and interdependent reality rather than as elements decreed by a sovereign deity. More freedom to choose and experience good necessarily means more freedom to make choices that lead to suffering. (If one could *only* choose "good," then it wouldn't be a choice, however good. While, surely, a universe in which *only* good exists would be lovely. But God cannot create unilaterally, so choice and freedom are inescapable qualities of the fabric of reality. This is important to remember when reflecting on the "meaning" of suffering in the lives of clients in spiritual distress.

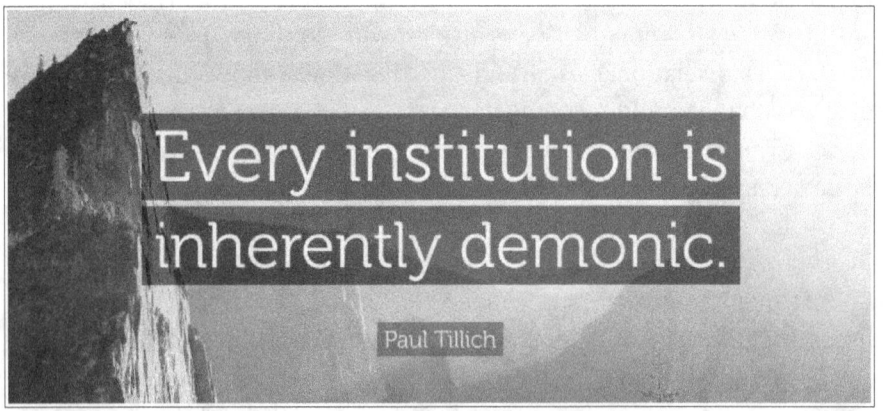

Every institution is inherently demonic.

Paul Tillich

Section III:
Dealing with Loss

In a culture that still too often denies the inevitability of death, it should come as no surprise that issues of loss, bereavement and grieving are the most common causes of spiritual distress. The fundamental human emotions have been summarized as "mad, sad, glad, scared" – "glad" rarely leads us to seek help, so "mad, sad, scared" are the basic feelings more likely to find their way into a consulting hypnotist's office. In all three, there is always an element of loss: one is angry at not getting what one wants (the loss of the longed-for) or at being treated badly (the loss of self-respect or the respect of others), one is sad (the feeling most often associated with the losses that lead obviously to grief), one is frightened (the loss of security, of safety, of the world one thought one had). Feelings of anger, sadness and fear are powerful. Allowed to fester without being used for insight, growth, wiser actions, they cause immense suffering, intense spiritual distress.

All faith traditions have their own ways of dealing with the meaning of suffering, grief and mortality, including the quest for non-attachment of Buddhism, the identification of suffering with redemption in Christianity, the hope of rebirth into a better life (in this world or another) in any number of belief systems, and the matter-of-fact acceptance in religious humanism, with hundreds of variations possible. The comfort and meaning offered by these doctrines, philosophies and hopes should not be underestimated. But they are very often just not enough.

Loss is painful – and not well understood.

In this section, we'll be considering several elements of the human experience of bereavement that will be helpful in working with clients in spiritual distress, including the universality of loss, specific factors that shape the experience of grief, the grieving process itself, and indications of problems in grieving and how to tell when a client's needs are beyond the normal scope of practice for a Consulting Hypnotist. We'll also be looking at some specific hypnotic techniques, metaphors, resources and a case study.

thankful for the sun on their bright petals
by Christian Skoorsmith (2023)

One of the secrets we do not know
as children is how many miscarried siblings
are buried in our backyards, under trees
alongside pets, surrounded still
by placentas that go on not being enough, still
holding in wholeness what would have been.

It takes years and many kid-free dinners
and bottles of wine before we discover how much
and how many of our friends have made quiet rest
in gardens, along hedges,
how many soft spots or sinkholes there.

Rest a moment ourselves in our own
feelings. We do not need to say
it was meant to be, in order to say
the loss no longer defines our lives, that flowers
have grown over those places, that we
are thankful for the sun on their bright petals.

The Universality of Loss

When speaking of bereavement and grief, it's natural to assume we are dealing with issues of dying and death. And of course we are – but the scope of loss is far wider than that. In addition to the spiritual challenge of grieving the end of life (actual or anticipated; others' or one's own), there are many other losses that can feel like a death: the loss of a job, of one's home, one's health, a relationship, a special object, a belief or ideal. While we will generally be speaking of loss as associated with death, do remember that there are many kinds of death. Anything that is valued and lost can be said to have died.

What other losses can you think of?
What is your own personal history of loss?
What do you yourself fear losing?

Few people talk easily about death, loss, bereavement – and our language can sometimes even be part of the problem. We speak of "losing" a loved one, for example, as though we had carelessly left them behind at a gas station. The carelessness associated by many with the word "loss" can make it seem that the bereaved is at fault. Unfortunately, especially with death, the greatest of all our losses, we seem to have no words that are any better. We have euphemisms ("passed over," "passed away," "went to heaven," "went to sleep," "bought the farm," "kicked the bucket," and so on) – phrases that act to shield us from the reality.

Yet every person blessed with awareness and relationships will also know that reality – that lives end, that situations change, that what we cherish today may not be with us tomorrow. Finding the spiritual strength to face those changes is rarely easy, but it can be facilitated by a deeper understanding of the nature of grief and the support of a caring, nonjudging listener and guide – such as you, the consulting hypnotist.

Such knowledge will not eliminate the pain – it may not even ease it, at least not as quickly as you and your client might wish. But if you are chosen to accompany another on the path of their grief, you are chosen not to paper over the suffering with platitudes or dismissals – as in the poem above, we do not need to say "it was meant to be" in order to say that it will not always be so close, so painful. In fact, silence is often a welcome testament to an understanding of suffering. As a Consulting Hypnotist, knowledge of the path can help the grieving client realize that their journey, while particular and specific to them, is also a universal one. It may take different forms, even different from what an individual expects for themselves, but healing is always possible.

Because grief is familiar to everyone, it is important that the consulting hypnotist be well aware of his or her own bereavement issues. Grief calls to grief, and it is all too easy to be overcome with sympathy for the pain being expressed, or worse, to be overcome by one's own remembered or anticipated griefs. Before you can guide others on their path to spiritual healing, see to the needs of your own spirit. Be sure you have the support you need to tend to your own journey. Don't let your own issues cloud your ability to help your client.

Factors Affecting the Grief Experience

The experience of grief is wide and varied, and we don't pretend to be able to cover all the nuances. We do hope to give you an idea of the kinds of questions you might ask and what to be listening for, in order to be helpful to someone who is suffering a wound that will never completely heal. This is important: grief never ends. We adapt to the reality of our losses; we are changed by the experiences and the ways in which we react and respond; but we are never truly "over" any painful loss.

It is human nature to expect that others will respond to life's changes and challenges the same way we would. That's rarely a wise approach, and when helping someone negotiate the journey of grief, it can be a harmful one.

This too is important: Short of behavior that is physically or emotionally harmful to self or others, any behavior arising from grief is within the range of "normal." And some of the harmful behaviors may, in some contexts, be "normal," too.

How does your family/culture/religious community approach grieving? What do you regard as "normal" grief behavior?

The list of factors that shape how we learn to experience and express our grief is long, and this listing is far from complete. Each of these general categories will have many sub-groupings. When listening to the story of a client's distress, among the factors to consider would be

• national culture

- regional culture
- ethnicity
- religion
- the griever's basic personality
- the griever's age, life experiences, grief history, now and at the time of the loss
- the nature of the loss (sudden? violent? anticipated? "natural"? self-chosen?)
- the degree of life disruption (physical, social, psychological) caused by the loss
- the level of acceptance of and sympathy for the loss in the griever's immediate circle of family and friends, faith community, and larger community
- the griever's responsibilities and responses at the time of the loss

What other characteristics, experiences, values, expectations would you add to this list?

Many griefs are belittled by the wider culture, which makes the process of finding healing and peace far more difficult than it needs to be. A large part of the caring listener's task is simply to hear and to affirm the reality of the grief, not to judge it, not to diminish it, and certainly not to condemn it.

The Grieving Process

Most of us are probably familiar with the concept of "the stages of grief," from the work of Elisabeth Kubler-Ross. The stages she described – denial, anger, bargaining, depression, and acceptance – can be useful in understanding a particular person's grief process. It's important to remember that there is no rigid, universal, unchanging framework of grief (a classic story among hospice workers is of the Kubler-Ross disciple seen standing over the bed of a patient, screaming "You can't die now! You haven't accepted it yet!"). Still, there is a widely recognized general pattern, and knowing what that pattern usually looks like can be helpful. Again, it will not lessen the pain. But contextualizing it can help one to believe that one might somehow survive it.

The most common phases of the grieving process are:
1. shock & numbness
2. reality-testing/"searching & yearning"
3. the full realization of the loss & full experience of the pain of grieving
4. healing and reinvesting in life

The first phase is most intense in the first couple of weeks following a loss. It can include a wide variety of physical symptoms and sensations and a wide range of behaviors, none of which are any indication of the actual depth of feeling. (Remember the many factors that can affect how grief is experienced and expressed.) These intense feelings and the protective numbness can diminish relatively quickly, but will often return with just as much intensity at anniversaries, holidays, in emotionally-charged settings, or sometimes for no discernible reason at all.

During "searching and yearning," the subconscious mind is preoccupied with the loss, testing its reality and hoping to discover that it didn't really happen after all. The fear of going crazy at this time is not uncommon – this is when people tend to hear their beloved's voice, see them in a favorite chair, pick up the phone to call them, carry around a favorite object or wear their clothing. Appetite changes, tearfulness, restlessness, sleep disruption, the sensation of "waves" of anguish are all common. This phase, because it is so non-rational, is not well understood nor regarded by the larger society with much sympathy. Queen Victoria was allowed to mourn Prince Albert for the rest her life, but parents who turn the bedroom of a dead child into a shrine are encouraged to seek professional help. During the months (and sometimes years, as these experiences can fade and then recur) of reality testing, the best help for the griever is compassionate support.

Eventually, the mind can no longer hold to the hope that the loss was an illusion, and the deepest pain of grief sets in. Restlessness gives way to apathy, personal care may be ignored, a sadness that seems impossible to lift grips the heart. Old patterns and activities are often abandoned because they no longer provide any meaning or comfort, and there is not yet any energy to help new patterns emerge. Again, there is very limited societal support or understanding, because by now – some 4 to 6 months after the loss and sometimes continuing several months longer – the rest of the world not immediately affected by that loss has gone back to its usual routines.

This is often the point at which well-meaning family and friends and medical professionals will suggest antidepressants. Unless you are licensed to practice medicine, this is a tricky situation, but the "medication temptation," while understandable, is rarely helpful. The journey of grief can be delayed, but it cannot be stopped. Medicating natural grief will only slow the process. As soon as the medication is stopped, the griever will be right were they were when their grieving was chemically interrupted.

But in time, the spirit does heal. Over time, we learn to integrate our losses with our ongoing lives; life is reorganized in a way that makes the loss not forgotten but bearable. New and adequate coping patterns arise. The level of emotional investment in the dead decreases, and more energy is available for new relationships with life.

Often there is a subjective experience – a dream, a daydream, an inner voice, a piece of music conveying a message or a special meaning – that gives the griever the sense of having received permission to move out of grieving and rejoin the world, to live again, as the best possible honoring of the deceased.

This healing occurs in bursts in all of the phases, but it increases most noticeably around the sixth month after the loss, and continues over the next six to eighteen months. It commonly takes about two years – two full cycles of significant anniversaries, holidays, seasonal changes and the like – for the survivor's life to find its new normalities and grow more accustomed to and accepting of the new realities of life.

The phases are not neat and orderly. They can appear and vanish and reappear unexpectedly; they may overlap; they may arise in different sequences or repeat themselves; sometimes a phase may be skipped altogether.

And sometimes people do get stuck, and may need some help in order to move on toward healing.

Problems in Grieving

Just a reminder of what you already know: Grief hurts, and grief lasts a life-time. Short of behaviors harmful to oneself or to others, just about anything can be normal in grieving.

Grief is the price we pay for opening ourselves to love, to connec-tions, and so of course we are overwhelmed by it. Most people, with a bit of help and some time, pass through the worst of grief's devastation. How do we recognize when someone (including ourselves) may be getting "stuck" in grief and so experiencing even more pain, even more disruption than their healing might require?

What are the signs of unhealthy grief?

1. an inability to accept the reality of the loss
2. an inability to recognize or to accept grieving behavior in oneself or in others
3. an inability to accept and adjust to changes in life that result from the loss
4. an inability to "let go" emotionally of the lost and reinvest that energy into ongoing life

In some extreme cases, professional intervention by a licensed ther-apist may be necessary. Such extremes, however, are rare. There is, in fact, reason to believe that grief is one life situation that does not usually benefit from explicitly therapeutic psychological or medical interventions. Grief is a dis-ease of the spirit, and rarely will any approach but the spiritual be of sig-nificant help.

Most of the time, what is needed is being with someone who is will-ing and able to listen in a sympathetic, nonjudgmental fashion, acknowledg-ing the reality of the pain and giving the griever support in finding and fol-lowing their own best path to healing. The greatest help comes through af-firmation of the reality of the loss, allowing the expression of the full range of feelings (not just anger or sorrow or fear, but also guilt, relief, confusion, and any number of others), helping the bereaved to see what is blocking their path to healing, and encouraging a loving releasing of that which is now gone in order to participate fully in the life that is still to come, all while gently reminding the griever that the journey of grief takes a long time, and there are no easy ways through it.

Additional Elements for Grief and Loss

We have already spent considerable time on the HOPE techniques for developing a Spiritual Profile of and Spiritual Goals for a client, and need not repeat that material here. We would simply add two additional considerations.

First, when doing the Spiritual Assessment, you will want to be listening for and eliciting your client's history of loss. When grief is the specific Spiritual Distress that has brought a client to you, you'll find it helpful to ask the same sorts of questions we looked at earlier: How have they been taught to grieve? What do they think "normal" grieving looks like? What are the losses have they have already suffered or fear they must face? What does their religious background tell them – whether they consciously believe it at present or not – about death?

Second, when considering the client's Spiritual Profile after your work has been successfully completed, remember that your client is seeking healing of his or her grief, but will never be completely healed. Success will be measured by the client's ability to reengage in life, to remember the dead or lost (when the grief is for a job, a faith, an identity, etc.) with honesty and compassion, and to go forward aware of the gifts the client has received, in spite of the pain of the process of grieving.

There are two specific brief techniques we offer for your consideration. Depending upon your goals for a particular induction, they may be used in several ways during the 5-part hypnotic process:

The Candles of Witness and Memory:

The Rev. Dr. Lindsay Bates, BCH, wrote this as a concluding ritual for memorial services. The actual candles are lit during reflective music at the beginning of the service. They are extinguished at the end, the first with a breath, the second between moistened fingertips [a glass of water is kept hidden in the pulpit; the congregation does not see the moistening]. She has since used this often in hypnotic work with the grieving.

In extinguishing the Candles of Witness and Memory,
we blow out one flame

to scatter into the wide universe
any remaining anger, hurt, disappointment;
to scatter and dismiss all that deserves to be forgotten.

And we enfold and so take within ourselves the other,
taking into ourselves
all that was good, all that was joyful, all that was loving;
taking and keeping within our own hearts
all that deserves to be kept.

The Forgiveness Script:

We first heard these words from the Rev. Randy Sawyer many years ago at an annual meeting of the National Association of Clergy Hypnotherapists; many others have written or adapted similar words.

For my own sake,
I forgive you
for everything you have done to me
real or imagined
I forgive you and set you free.
And in setting you free
I set myself free
for health and happiness

The hypnotic experience for grief work follows the same 5 steps as all other Spiritual Hypnotism, with some additional elements:

1. Remember and experience the Mystery and the Beauty of the universe, despite its times of hardship and sorrow.

2. Focus on the goodness manifest in the client's life and the promise of healing.

3. Guide the client to reflect upon their grief and a particular issue within it, using both words and appropriate silence for the client to do their own inner work. You might suggest a healing encounter with the beloved dead in a safe and peaceful place, and help the client have the conversation they need for healing.

You might guide a revisiting of the funeral or memorial service so that the words the client needed to hear may be heard. You might invite a meeting with a spiritually significant figure (one you suggest, based upon your knowledge of your client's beliefs, or letting the image arise from their own deeper self), who will offer compassion, wisdom and peace. If there are issues of forgiveness, you might invite the client to imagine writing down all the things that need to be released, and then, as that list is burned or buried or entrusted to an angel or a great eagle who carries it up to the Sun – whatever image will speak to your client's beliefs – you might invite the client to imagine him or herself speaking the words of the Forgiveness Script above.

4. Lift up the vision of a future already coming into being, of increasing peace and acceptance, of a lifting of the burden of pain and a return of more and more healing and joy-filled memories. You might use future pacing to guide your client along the path of grief, as appropriate to wherever they are in their journey, as a reassurance that they are on a healing path. Always assume and affirm that the journey of grieving, though difficult, will lead ultimately to a place of comfort, acceptance, healing and peace.

5. Use the Master's Voice to offer an appropriate autosuggestion based upon what is most likely to help your client move forward on the path of grieving and healing: "Josie, your mother understands, and she wants you to be happy." "Kim, your father is proud of you and the courage you show in your life." "Jennie, you have a loving heart, and sharing your compassion with others brings comfort to you."

In Summary

You can help your clients find their own path through their grieving – find the meaning and the comfort and the acceptance that will allow them to move forward with their own lives – but the path is theirs to walk. We are changed by our losses. Our challenge is to find ways to become more whole in a different way, that honors our loves, our losses, and our own precious lives.

Resources

There are hundreds – probably thousands – of books, journals, articles, websites and support groups available to help those who are grieving and those who are supporting grievers in their journeys. Some of the books you may have to hunt for, but most are easily found. And one web site will quickly lead to many dozens of others!

The Compassionate Friends
 the United States http://www.compassionatefriends.org/
 Canada http://www.tcfcanada.net/
 Great Britain http://www.tcf.org.uk/

Friedman, Dayle A., ed. *Jewish Pastoral Care: A Practical Handbook from Traditional & Contemporary Sources* (2ⁿᵈ edition, 2005)

Grollman, Earl A. *Living When a Loved One Has Died* (Beacon Press, 1997)
       (ed.) *What Helped Me When My Loved One Died* (Beacon Press,1982)
       (ed.) *Explaining Death to Children* (Beacon Press, 1967)
       (ed.) *Concerning Death: A Practical Guide for the Living* (Beacon
       Press, 1974, Beacon)
Rabbi Grollman has written and/or edited a number of books on bereavement issues, and most are available in updated editions.

Hospice http://www.hospicenet.org/
       http://www.hospicefoundation.org/

Kirkwood, Neville A. *A Hospital Handbook on Multiculturalism & Religion* (revised ed., 2005)

Kubler-Ross, Elisabeth. *On Death & Dying* (1969)
       Questions & Answers on Death & Dying (1974)

Magida, Arthur J. & Matlins, Stuart M., eds. *How to Be a Perfect Stranger: A Guide to Etiquette in Other People's Religions* (hardcover, 2 volumes, 1996/97; paperback 4ᵗʰ edition, 2006)

Matlins, Stuart M., ed. *The Perfect Stranger's Guide to Funerals and Grieving Practices: A Guide to Etiquette in Other People's Religious Ceremonies* (Skylight Paths Publishing, 2000)

Moore, Thomas, *Care of the Soul in Medicine: Healing Guidance for the Patients, Families, and the People Who Care for Them* (Hay House Inc., 2nd edition, 2011)

Survivors of Suicide   http://www.survivorsofsuicide.com/
    http://www.suicidology.org/index.cfm

Westberg, Granger E. *Good Grief* (a frequently-reissued classic, originally published in 1962).

Worden, J. William. *Grief Counseling & Grief Therapy: A Handbook for the Mental Health Professional* (3rd edition, 2001)

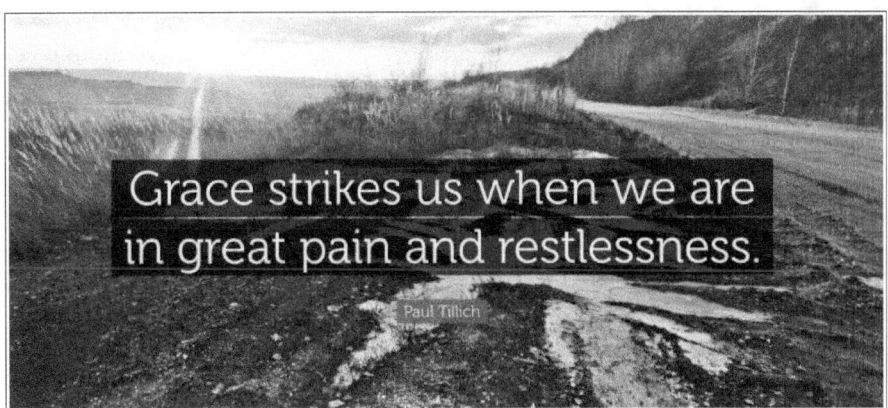

Accelerated Grief Process
By Celeste Hackett

The following was not part of the original 2007 curriculum. It is, however, a valuable technique to have at the ready – either as a standalone practice or as backup method should the client persistently experience the "bad grief" described above. This is a specialized application of parts therapy, sometimes called gestalt therapy or even chair therapy. As such, it is versatile and intuitive, can be led by the hypnotist but deeply relies on the client's conscious and unconscious participation. It, therefore, respects the client's own spiritual/religious beliefs while at the same time offering a directive approach the hypnotist can actively use. In keeping with the manualized format of this book, Celeste Hackett has broken the process down into step-by-step instructions and supplied helpful vignettes and script-lets to make the work clearer.

If you want to be truly happy in life, you will have to master the art of letting go. And when you consider all the losses you've already had in your life, you should be pretty good at it by now. No one gets through life without sorrow. Losses begin for us as babies and seem to grow as we do. We have no choice in the matter. We will think we have something, or someone, relax into the idea of forever and then, one day the inevitable happens. There is only the question of when.

Letting go of people who are important to us can be particularly challenging, but after observing how clients move into radically positive changes after devastating losses again and again, I want to make two, perhaps startling, points. 1) Grieving is actually very, very good for you. And 2) We, as hypnotists, should *reconsider* any beliefs that encouraging clients to grieve a loss *forever* is in any way acceptable. The goal for our grieving clients should be the end of "bad" feelings associated with the loss, so that they can embrace optimistically, the next chapter, whatever it may be.

Now, don't worry, I am not saying that you should shame your clients for taking the time to feel the emotions associated with loss. That is part of moving through grief. I am just saying that to *refrain* from raising or exploring this idea, and then *not* suggesting that the pain of their grief can come to an end, is doing them a disservice.

Before I move on, if you are still grieving something, I am aware this may not sit well with you. If this is the case, you might even get mad at me for saying this. That is understandable. When you are ready, read on. There is much you can do for yourself if the desire to be free from grief arises. You can apply the techniques written here for example. Also, if you want to stay where you are, that is fine too, but I am not going to be *that* person, the one who tells you that you must keep suffering. Doing that would keep you from feeling and becoming something even more amazing than you have ever felt or been. I don't want you to miss that.

CAN GRIEF BE GOOD FOR YOU?

So, how *can* grief possibly be good for you? Well, most of us live as if there is no end to our time on earth. That works for a while, and maybe it's meant to be that way, but it's simply not the truth. There is no doubt that the harsh reality of physical life being impermanent is tough to accept. It has been said that the truth hurts and in the case of loss that is undeniably correct. However, there is another saying that will allow us to fight this fire with fire, and it is that the *truth sets us free*. Look, we all must grow up sometime or remain in ignorance. The latter, at best, will beget a sort of becoming numb or -stagnant; at worst, it will cause continued suffering, especially when other inevitable losses layer themselves upon each other.

REALIZATIONS ARE THE KEY TO LETTING GO

There are several stages of grief that people go through as this book mentions. Each stage requires realizing something important before being able to move on to the next. Given the time, most people will go through these stages needing no help at all, but others get stuck and that is where a little help will be appreciated. Your primary job will be to help your clients achieve realizations that move them toward acceptance, peace and finally optimism and hope. To do this you can use any technique that works. Great ones have already been given in this book. This chapter offers its own set of techniques and ideas for you.

You may be wondering about the realizations that move clients through grief. What are they? Some will be unique to your client, but most of them just make up the normal process of letting go. Realizing, for instance, that a loved one is not coming back can help profoundly. The process of accepting that can be very painful, but once done, eventually, peace rises. However, you don't have to make peace come – it has been there all along. You are just facilitating the removal of any ideas or emotions that have been covering it up. It is comforting to know that each realization in the grief process will bring more peace to your client. In fact, they will become much more stable and mature and their understanding of life itself will profoundly and beautifully change for them.

ABOUT THIS GRIEF PROCESS – WHO IS THE IDEAL CLIENT?

I call the process that I use "Accelerated Grief Process" (or AGP) because that's what it does. It accelerates a process already in motion by moving clients along more quickly. I learned about it from Cal Banyan initially when he did a brief outline of it in a training class, but I am not sure who originated it. Through discussions about grief work with other hypnotists and applying what I learned with clients over the years, I was inspired to add more to those original techniques.

When you use this process, keep in mind that if your client's loss is very recent you may have to repeat it more than once before they experience total resolution. These clients may benefit from time between sessions. I like to let them set the pace. That said, even a client whose loss is coming from the most horrifying circumstances, will usually find a good deal of relief in just one session, if applied properly. This may not be a complete resolution yet, but it will help them to be more functional, which is a good step in the right direction.

Another type of client for this process is someone who really wants to get over their grief and knows they must. Many times, this is the client whose very survival or the survival of their family is being affected by their grief. An example would be a businessman who can't depend on himself to be emotionally stable in meetings and therefore finds himself avoiding them, putting his livelihood in jeopardy. This type of client has usually already been grieving for many weeks, months and sometimes years, and does not need anyone to point out the toll grief is taking.

You may also find unresolved grief keeping your clients from achieving a goal when you are working with them for entirely other things such as weight loss, procrastination, or overcoming any variety of fears. In these cases, when unresolved grief is found, just detour into this process. After the grief has been dealt with, give suggestions that your client can now do or become what they want. It really is that simple.

One important thing to know about working with clients who are grieving is that sadness, usually expressed by the words "I miss you," is the most common emotion that must be resolved. However, it isn't the only emotion that can cause clients to hold on to grief. All "negative" emotions (feelings that don't feel good) relating to the one who has passed should be resolved. If not, the grief may continue in one form or another. The top feelings that cause grief to go unresolved are sadness, anger, and guilt. So, at least make sure that you address these three. Here is the outline.

Accelerated Grief Process (Basic Outline)

STEP ONE: Induce and deepen hypnosis. It is not necessary, nor even necessarily the best practice, to bring your client to deep relaxation when you do this work. If you do that clients can slip into aphasia and have a hard time talking. We need them to be alert enough to talk and to feel their feelings. (Hypnosis is not relaxation, of course.)

Note, if your client is in hypnosis when working on something else and you realize they have unresolved grief standing in the way of their changes, just detour from what you are doing to step two.

STEP TWO: Have your client imagine the dead. You can set up a special scene. Ideas are:
- The beach
- The forest
- The kitchen at home
- In a quiet church with candles
- In a hospital bed

Example: "And now I wonder if you could imagine walking on a beautiful nature trail in the forest. It's a lovely day. The birds are singing. You feel a nice breeze as you walk and after a while you find a bench

along the trail to sit on. As you are enjoying the peace of nature all
around you, you notice you aren't the only one on the trail today. In
the distance you see a woman walking toward you. As she gets nearer
you notice there is something familiar in her walk, and now you real-
ize, it's your mother. She has come back to help you out."

Be prepared for tears or the struggle to hold them in. This is a
process, so don't rush it. Relax and be *with* your client. A lot of this work is
about just being willing to take the time to be there with them as they go
through it. Another very important aspect of AGP is to ask questions to gen-
erate realizations that provide relief. (You can find examples of these kinds
of questions in steps 5 and 6.) Other than that, your job is to *cheerlead* the
expression of emotions and draw their attention to them. This helps them to
feel and let emotions out, so that afterwards, their natural inner peace becomes evident. To help them release feelings you can use phrases such as:

"That's right. Let it out."
"It's feels good to cry at a time like this."
"It's okay to cry. Anybody would."
"Oh my, I can see your heart is so full of sadness."

Do not make the mistake of sending a message that leads them to
hold feelings *in*. For instance, watch your tone. *You* may be surprised at how
much you just want to say to them, *"Uh, it's okay,"* while patting their arm.
The meta-message that they may take from that being: "*Please stop it. You
are making me uncomfortable.*" Also, think hard before you hand them a tis-
sue. This can also be taken as: *"You're done now, stop it. Wipe those tears
away. Pull yourself up; let's dry them and get on to feeling happy. You're
killing me."*

All of this leads to another point: Work on your own feelings. Because if their emotions are making you uncomfortable, this only means that
some of your subconscious feelings are not healed and are being triggered
by their expression of feeling. When you are emotionally balanced you can
stay neutral and do this job much more effectively.

STEP THREE: Encourage your client to say whatever needs to be said to the
dead, so they can finally be at peace with their passing. Also, continue to encourage the release of feelings (crying etc.).

Example: "*Inside of you are the words you need to say to finally be at peace with your mom's passing. Talk to her now.*"

STEP FOUR: Have them "be" the dead and respond *as* their mother.

Example: "*Good. Be your mother. Mom, respond to what you just heard. Your daughter thinks it was her fault that you died (for example). What do you have to say to that?*"

STEP FIVE: Go back and forth between your client talking and the deceased talking. You can also ask questions of both deceased and your client to help move things along.

Examples for Mom:
"*Why didn't you tell her you were sick, Mother?*"
"*She thinks it is her fault that you died, is that true?*"
"*Is there anything she could have done to save you?*"
"*Mom, are you in any pain now?*"
"*Do you want your daughter to continue suffering?*"
"*What do you want for her life now that you are gone?*"

When the deceased says something that may be comforting you can ask your client, "*How does that make you feel?*" Feel free to go back and forth between the client and the dead.

Examples for your client:
'*Your mother says it was just her time to go. Respond to that.*"
"*Your mom says she doesn't want you to hold on to sadness, but to have a happy life. How does that make you feel?*"
"*Maybe it's just me, but you still seem so sad. Is that true? Then, tell her how much you miss her.*"
"*Tell your mother what you miss about her most.*"

When you or your client are at a loss for words you can always say: "*Inside of you (mom or client) are the words that need to be said (to feel better, to find peace, to forgive, to let go of sadness or for our daughter to feel better, find peace etc.). Speak to your daughter," or "talk to your mom from your heart now."*

Be prepared that you may have to help your client express anger or other emotions that talking back and forth like this doesn't relieve. If you haven't already learned a process of forgiveness or working with guilt, fear etc., it is time to do so. (I give some ideas below.) Know that you may have to shift into those processes along the way so that guilt, fear, anger, and so on, do not derail the grief/release.

STEP SIX: Final words.

> *Example*:
>
> *"Mom, do you have any final words of wisdom or encouragement for your little girl?*
>
> *"Will she see you again? What will it be like then? What will it be like to be together again?"*
>
> *"Will you always send your love from where you are?"*
>
> *"How do you want her life to be from here on?"*
>
> *"How would you like her to remember you? I mean, you looked terrible when you were sick. Is this how you want her to remember you?"*

That last question can give your client a new parting image of the deceased instead of the traumatizing view in the casket, or having found them dead, or bloated with tubes coming out of them in the hospital.

STEP SEVEN: Check for changes. *"Now how do you feel about your mom's passing?"* If you get "peaceful," "relieved," "better," or something to that effect, you can move to Step Eight.

However, if you don't perceive that a positive shift has happened, you may encourage "Mom" to find another way she would like to be remembered or there could be another problem to find out what it is, just ask. *"If you don't feel better, what do you feel?"* Usually, resolution comes from fully expressing whatever the feeling that is left.

The top three feelings that get in the way of clients resolving grief are: sadness, anger, and guilt. What follows is a dialog technique to work with each of those feelings when they are still present and preventing the client from making progress. (You may have to engage in this kind of dialog with the client throughout AGP. AGP is not merely suggesting things to your client. It keeps you on your toes.)

Examples of Dialogues in AGP

Sadness

When the client says "I am still sad," this means they haven't cried enough or said enough about how sad they are. More expression is needed. Sad in this example is about the literal loss of her mother. She needs to be encouraged to say again and again while feeling it inside: "I miss you so much! I will never see you again! I am so sad!"

Feeling and then speaking reduces the feelings. There is an old saying, "if you can feel it, you can heal it." This is definitely true for this process. If your client can not find the words you can give them to her.

Example:
Client: *No, I still feel bad!*

Hypnotist: *What is that bad feeling? Sadness? Guilt? Anger? Or Something else?*

Client: *I think I am still so sad!*

Hypnotist: *Okay, tell your mother how much you miss her.*

Client: *Mom! I miss you so much.*

Hypnotist: *Good say it again from the depths of your heart. Tell her how much you are hurting! Let all of your feelings out. Inside of you are the words that need to be said so you can be at peace with your mom's passing.*

Client: *Mom! Mom! Why did you leave me? I am so sad. I miss you so much!*

Keep this up until you see or suspect a shift in your client. Then, ask again: How do you feel now? If there is still sadness, repeat. You can also use the Pillow Trick and/or EFT (explained below).

For sadness there is another thing you can do. Since you cannot ever replace a person and sadness is the feeling most closely related to loss, try having them replace what that person brought into their life.

Replacing What Was Lost

Hypnotist: *Your mother sounds like a wonderful person. Tell me, what did she bring into your life? In other words, what was so great about her?*

Client: *My mother was someone that was always encouraging to me. She could be relied upon for babysitting my children. I trusted her. She had the most beautiful voice. She made me laugh and see things from a different perspective. Most of all, she was always there when I needed her.*

Hypnotist: *All right then. Let's take a look at it. Let's talk to mom about this. Be Mom. Mother, your daughter is in so much pain and is struggling to move on. Can you tell her who can she look to now for encouragement, and who will always be there for her?*

Client-as-Mom: *Oh honey, you know you can look to your husband! He loves you so much. And you can look to God.*

Hypnotist: *Who can she trust to babysit her children?*

Mom: *Your sister can help you with that and your friend Debbie. She loves the kids. And don't forget God is watching over them too.*

Hypnotist: *What will she ever do without your beautiful voice?*

Mom: *Honey, my voice will always be in your heart and mind forever. All you have to do is think of me and you'll hear me say the things I always used to say to you, like how glad I am to have you for a daughter. Also, you can look to your sister. Doesn't she sound a lot like me? It's time for you to lean on each other. You'll grow closer now.*

Hypnotist: *OK one last thing mother, who can make her laugh and see things from different perspectives?*

Mom: *That would be her brother Nicholas!*

Hypnotist: *OK client, you heard from your mother now how do you feel?*

Client: *Better! Thank you, mom! I love you so much!*

Hypnotist: *Great, on a scale of one to 10, with 10 being the grief we started off with and zero being none at all, where are you?*

Client: *About a 2.*

Hypnotist: *Great. Let's move on.*

From here move to Step Eight.

Anger

When your client says they are still feeling bad and that the "bad" feeling is anger, you'll have to find a way of getting forgiveness of the deceased. How do you do that? Any way your training has taught you to come to forgiveness. If you are adept at Emotional Freedom Technique (EFT or "Tapping"), then do that. If your specialty is Neuro-Linguistic Programming (NLP), you may find working in sub-modalities and reframing to be successful. If you are trained in Five-Phase Advanced Transformational Hypnosis (5-PATH®), utilizing Forgiveness of Others (FOO) would be natural. You get the idea.

That having been said, you may very well not need *any* of that stuff to get forgiveness of the deceased. Why? I don't know exactly why, but it truly is easier to get forgiveness of the dead than the living.

I can guess why. It seems like it could be any of these reasons:

- Clients just want to go easy on a person who has died. Clients feel so sorry for them because they died.

- To be mad at the dead may be a taboo that runs very deep: you just don't speak ill of the dead. So, how could you be angry at them?

- Some clients believe that when you die you become an angel. Who can be mad at an angel?

- Some clients think the person's death is enough to forgive them as it pays off any "debt" to the client.

- Some clients think that, as mad/hurt as they are, they do not want their loved one to go to hell. What if God hears them complain? God might take that seriously and judge them too harshly.

The truth is, though, we don't have to know. We can ask clients themselves! I am going to start asking my grief clients if the deceased is easier to forgive, now that they are "gone," and why. I'll let you know what I find.

Example of how to get forgiveness within AGP:

Client: *I still feel bad! I think I am angry at my mom!*

Hypnotist: *Tell her what she did to hurt you. She is listening.*

Client: *Mom, you always loved my brother Nicholas best! It was so obvious. That really hurt me. You even bought him a new car when he graduated from high school. You never did that for me!*

Depending on how strong the anger is I may take out the pillow and have them hit it as per the pillow trick below. Once I sense a shift in them, I move to mom.

> Hypnotist: *Mom! How could you do that? You really hurt (client)!*
> *What kind of a mother does that?"*

I am going to go after the deceased somewhat harshly, so that my client wants to protect her. It's hard to be angry at someone and want to protect them at the same time. Remember, in my world, forgiveness means no longer being angry at them.

> Client-as-Mom: *Oh honey, I know I did that. I just couldn't help it. He*
> *was my baby and I just wasn't through wanting to be a mom.*
> *I loved you as much. When you were born your older sister*
> *was jealous of you too. I have always loved babies so much.*
> *Please forgive me.*

> Hypnotist: *She seems sorry. You have kids. Maybe you can understand*
> *some of her feelings. She said she was sorry too. Do you be-*
> *lieve her?*

> Client: *Yes, I do! She loved me so much. I see that now.*

> Hypnotist: *Can you forgive her for that?*

> Client: *Yes. I really can.*

> Hypnotist: *Are you angry about anything more? If so, tell her.*

In this way, you can go back and forth getting forgiveness on every offense that stands in the way of your client feeling better. Keep repeating until your client feels they have forgiven 100 percent, if possible. Feel free to weave in your own forgiveness/anger techniques if needed. Then, once complete, move to step eight.

Guilt

If your client reports still feeling bad at any point, and the feeling is guilt on their part, the good news is that it is one of the easiest feelings to get resolution on. Read the following exchange and you will get the idea.

> Hypnotist: *You say you still feel bad. Can you tell if you are more sad, angry, guilty or something else?*

> Client: *I just feel so bad that we had a fight on the phone that morning. I can't stop thinking about it.*

Clients cannot always name their feelings, so sometimes you have to read between the lines. What the client is saying indicates guilt.

> Hypnotist: *Mother, do you hear what she is saying. She feels terrible. She has been thinking of her words since she heard you passed. Mother, please help her to feel better. Speak to your daughter.*

> Client-as-Mom: *Listen to me dear, mothers and daughters don't always see eye to eye. And honestly, I have always loved how feisty you are. I love you so much and I know you love me too. Our love goes beyond space and time and petty arguments. Please do not do this to yourself.*

> Hypnotist: *Client, how does that make you feel?*

> Client: (wiping tears) *Much better.*

From here you can try moving to Step Eight.

STEP EIGHT: Have your client say a productive good-bye so they can finally be at peace with mom's passing. This is especially important for the client who laments that they never got to say goodbye.

> <u>Example</u>: *Now that you are feeling better and you know that _____ (mom is at peace etc.), it is time to say goodbye. Inside of you are the words to say goodbye that will bring you peace with mom's passing.*

Afterwards, ask them if they are ready to let mom go. If not, go back to earlier steps of speaking to mom and listening to mom (STEPS 3 AND 4). Then try again. Keep repeating until your client is "at peace with mom's passing."

This whole process is about expressing, processing, and finally letting go mentally, physically, and emotionally. This is the *natural grief process* in a nutshell but sped up for modern times. Most people, these days, give merely a nod to the part of the process that once required unrestrained emoting, screaming, questioning, and grappling with those questions. AGP gives us a way to honor this tried-and-true means of change but helps to accelerate it for our more fast-paced world.

STEP NINE: Double check that your client has changed by asking them to think about a date in the future that, *in the past*, would have been difficult for them to deal with.

> *Example*: *Good. Now that you have said good-bye (let Mom go), let's move into the future. Now, it is Christmas this year. Mom is not there. How do you feel?*

If your client still has a lot of emotions go back to steps 3 and 4 and repeat.

You can always gauge the amount of grief by asking *"if your grief was at a 10 when we started and zero is no grief at all, where are you now?"* Depending on what has occurred in the session, the time this has taken, and the type of client in my chair, I may go for zero or level 1, 2 or 3. If I leave any grief in place, I will schedule a follow up.

STEP TEN: When your client can think of Mom's passing in a peaceful, calm way and they say they feel much better (or something like that) then you are ready to do reinforcement suggestions for continuing to feel this way. You can have the deceased hug your client, if appropriate, or say final words of encouragement as well.

> *Example*: *Is it okay if Mom gives you a hug before she goes back to where she came from? Good. Mom, give your daughter a warm, loving embrace.* (Pause to give them a little time together.)

Some hypnotists say that we should not allow the deceased to "always be with" the client. If the client or client-as-deceased expresses any desire for continued presence, instead suggest to the deceased: *"You cannot stay, but you can send your love from where you are. How does that sound?"* Such hypnotists don't want the deceased haunting the client, which then moves into the realm of spiritual attachment and releasement work. If this aligns with your thinking, this would be the opportune moment to have the "spirit" of the dead send love from where they are (up in the heavens for example). Even if you do not think like this, I would advise making these suggestions anyway, for the ongoing relief of the client. But that's just me.

After the hug, I like to suggest that Mom turns and goes back to where she came from. I usually ask my client how Mom looks as she leaves. My clients usually say, *"She looks happy,"* or *"She is floating, smiling and all in white,"* or *"She is going to grandpa. They both look so happy!"* This subconsciously goes with my client into her future, but I may suggest *"and now this is how you will always remember her."*

STEP 11: Make suggestions of how clients will benefit from the resolved grief. This will be personal for each client.

> *Example*: *Now that you know your mother is happy and you feel free of guilt and sadness you are going to find that your energy returns. Because your emotions are balanced, you feel stronger. You can conduct meetings now with confidence. And you no longer need to eat sugar to distract from those feelings because they are gone now. You feel so much better. So much lighter and so much happier.*

STEP 12: Test out the suggestions by taking your client into the future, one more time, to a time when in the past their grief would have caused a problem. See if the changes made in the grief work have also changed how they feel and handle what would've bothered them before.

> *Example*: (In the case of the businessman) *At the count of 3 you decide to conduct a much-needed meeting. It's time to begin talking, 1,2, 3. How do you feel?*

If they report they feel better give suggestions that reinforce that such as *"Good and now you will find that meetings are easy and you are back to your old self, even better."*

If they do not give a good report either the grief process wasn't completed or there are other feelings causing the future to be problematic. In the latter case, just move into whatever process you normally would use to uncover what is causing that and to remedy that problem.

If you feel there is more grief work to do you can detour back with *"at the count of one, Mom is back to help you again 3-2-1. Now, tell her* (for example) *I am still sad mom, and it is hurting me."* Repeat step 3 and the others again until you learn that your client's future has improved due to the grief work. Give direct suggestions to reinforce.

Feel good about yourself and happy for your client and emerge them.

A NOTE ON CLIENTS LETTING FEELINGS OUT

The phrases given to encourage expression of feelings may need to be used throughout this process, especially when clients are struggling to hold feelings in. These phrases are just examples, of course. The main thing is to come from your heart and *encourage* emotional expression.

You may also have to educate your client a bit directly and push a bit, especially if they are struggling hard in order to stifle them. You can say something like:

> *Look, Jane, the whole world might have told you not to cry and to just get over it because grief just isn't encouraged in our society, but if you keep that up you might never_____(lose weight, stop smoking, be able to conduct that business meeting with confidence, be there for your children, or whatever they say the grief is causing). Your subconscious is bringing these feelings up to be released and knows you have found a safe place to do that. Let it out, so you can feel better and _____(get what she wants). Just do it. Come on now. It's going to feel so good to let it out.*

Some clients have a particularly tough time letting feelings out. Some don't need to because for them to talk about it is enough. This is rare though, so don't settle for that right away. Push a little or even a lot if you think that they need it. If you push with love they won't mind.

THE PILLOW TRICK

One of the most useful tools for clients who stifle feelings is a pillow. I don't know why, but once they start hitting a pillow the tears begin to flow. They can't hold them in anymore. You can transition to the pillow this way:

> *I'm going to put a pillow on your lap. (place pillow on lap) Now, I want you to make two fists and begin hitting the pillow. As you do, say what you are feeling such as "I miss you so much mom"! Come on. You can do it.*

DON'T LIKE THE PILLOW?

This is an excellent place to do EFT. *"Even though I can't express my feelings, I just want to hold them in...," "Even though I don't want to hit the pillow...," "Even though I feel stupid or embarrassed doing this...."* You can even alternate between having the client hit the pillow and EFT.

Almost everyone knows what Emotional Freedom Technique is, so I won't give an explanation. If you are unfamiliar with it, free training is widely available. Just google it and watch a video or take an on-line class. Like any useful tool or technique used outside of hypnosis it works even better with clients who are *in* hypnosis.

WORKING WITH ESPECIALLY DIFFICULT CLIENTS

Over the years there have been occasions where I could not make headway with a client because of something I couldn't see or understand. You will run into your limitations and those of clients in situations like this. Whether it is a grief client or some other client I am trying to help, I have found that the best thing I can do is *to keep at it.* Where most hypnotists re-fer clients out or, as some say, *"fire them,"* I most often don't. I dig deeper.

If everything points to them *not* being mentally ill or having some other something that I can't really help with, taking on an attitude of unre-lenting interest, curiosity, love, plus the intention to figure it out no matter what, will, in the long run, serve both of us best. For me, this means I leave no soldier behind. I will see clients at much reduced rates, even for free if I must. Why? Because these are the clients that teach. I mean obviously, I am missing something. I want to learn what it is. Plus, the glory of change is so pronounced after such trials. It just feels so good.

I didn't' always do it this way. I referred out like everybody else, but what can I say? I love people who puzzle me. I used to get all worked up, trying *hard* in these cases. That was stressful, so I don't do that anymore. I just ask them questions, give them time, and wait to be inspired. I also trust that "Something" will help if I just keep with it. Something is my name for God at these moments.

This is why I gave up my state licensed school. I saw so many hypnotists teaching with so little knowledge. I wanted to get good at *doing the work*. The struggle with my own ego has been very worth it. It was a struggle because, like everyone speaking of losses, I hate to fail.

Don't worry. There is enough here to help you and with a little ingenuity and your own unrelenting attitude of sticking with it, *Something* will guide you, too. Hasn't that always been there for you anyway? Enjoy the people who puzzle you.

WRAPPING IT ALL UP

In closing, I'd like to share something with you. When I was a child and I became afraid of death for the first time, I nervously asked my dad, *"What happens to us when we die?"* He simply said, *"Well, Dear, death is just a part of life."* It wasn't so much what he said, but his peaceful acceptance of death that has carried me through many losses over the years. In his own way he let me know that there was nothing to worry about.

Our own death is the last loss. We never know what it is going to be like, but I have noticed each loss I encounter just brings me more freedom. This is the power of practicing the art of letting go. Working through our losses and even preparing for our own death are integral parts of being able to help clients walk the journey through their losses. Who doesn't want freedom? This may be the gift waiting for your clients at the end of their time with you.

There is faith in every serious doubt, namely, the faith in the truth as such, even if the only truth we can express is our lack of truth.

Paul Tillich

Section IV:
Death Preparation Exercises

If spirituality is the human response to being alive and having to die, then every hypnotist who undertakes Spiritual Hypnotism needs to come to terms with the inevitability of their own death.

Drawing upon training exercises common in the hospice movement we present two exercises. The first is an exercise that the practitioner can do to come to terms with his or own mortality. The second is an exercise that might be used as part of the work with a dying client to help him or her pass with dignity and grace.

For the practitioner: Begin by inducing yourself into a hypnotic state using a favorite technique. Then:

1. Deepen the state by reflecting on the awe and power of our universe;
2. Reflect on the possibility for goodness that our universe provides;
3. Reflect in silence on the key events and stepping-stones of your life so far; and
4. Imagine the world as it will be when you are no longer alive (it can be helpful to imagine the places you often go, and to notice that you are not there).
5. Finally, formulate and silently repeat to yourself a simple sentence that states what good you have done in the world during your lifetime. In this step, use the Master's Voice technique to refer to yourself in the third-person.

As an example, the fifth step of this procedure might be a sentence along the lines of "Alice always made others feel welcome, and did her best to be honest and kind." This exercise is a version of the "grave marker" exercise common in hospice training.

For a client: Begin by inducing the client into trance using any appropriate technique (for a client facing imminent death, you might want not to ask them to close their eyes – use an eye fixation or "soft eyes" suggestion and allow them to keep their eyes open or closed, as they prefer). Then:

1. Deepen the state by reflecting on the beauty and power of the universe;
2. Guide the client to reflect on the possibilities for good that exist;
3. Allow the client to spent time in silence reflecting on his or her life; and
4. Encourage the client to remember only good times from childhood to the present time.
5. Finally, ask the client to repeat the auto-suggestion "[Client name] is a good person whose life has brought goodness and joy to the world."

Encourage the client to adopt this method as a self-care exercise. The idea is to fill the mind with memories of what has been good and pleasant about life. This exercise is an extension of the Buddhist technique of facilitated dying. In Buddhist circles it is known as "watering the seeds of happiness so the seeds of unhappiness do not grow."

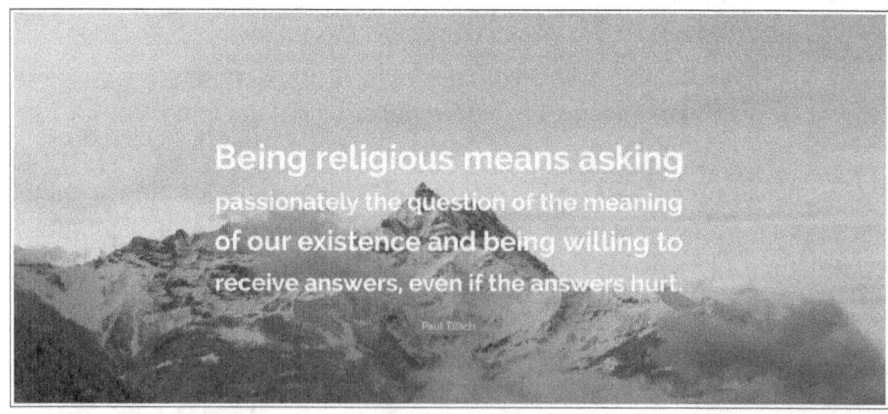

Being religious means asking passionately the question of the meaning of our existence and being willing to receive answers, even if the answers hurt.

Paul Tillich

Section V:
Spiritual Healing

There is much written about Spiritual Healing. The clergy who created this curriculum make a new contribution to this literature based upon our practical experience in the use of hypnotism for spiritual purposes.

We do not intend to take anything away from other systems of healing, such as Healing Touch, Therapeutic Touch, Reiki or other systems of energy work that function by the ancient ritual of the laying-on of hands. In many cases we ourselves embrace and practice such methods.

Our contribution here is to offer one more tool that a hypnotist might use to assist a client who seeks healing for him or herself, or for someone else.

In presenting this method we wish to acknowledge the contribution of hypnotist James M. Hoover who first devised the notion of Centrum, which is basic to our method here. We are using it in a way that Mr. Hoover did not intend, but wish to give him credit for the original idea upon which we have built.

The Healing of the Client

When the client presents him or herself for healing, our work is simply an extension of the five-part method already described:

1. The client is hypnotized, then the trance is progressively deepened by reflection on the awe and mystery of the universe;
2. the possibilities for good that creates;
3. a period of silence as the client reflects upon the need for a physical or emotional healing;

4.   a time when the client visualizes what a healing might do for the client, and finally

5.   the hypnotist, using the Master's Voice, delivers an auto-suggestion regarding the desired healing.

The Healing of a Person not Physically Present

A much more complex procedure is needed when the hypnotist wishes to help a person who is not a client or who is not physically present with the hypnotist. In this case the hypnotist will hypnotize him or herself and will deliver the auto-suggestion in the fifth step as a healing suggestion for the person who is not present.

Another suggestion is that clients can also be guided to do this as part of their own healing, on the theory that wishing good for others can help bring healing to oneself? This is a practice with a rich tradition in Buddhist thought reflecting an expanding care for all creatures.

However, we have found it helpful to introduce a new technique into the process when undertaking this particular form of Spiritual Hypnotism.

Centrum

The word "centrum" is simply Latin for "center." It is possible to think about the human personality as a collection of parts. Each part represents an aspect of our personality from time past. At different times these different parts activate and speak with a louder voice in the "town meeting" of our minds.

For example, one of the writers of this curriculum might list his "parts" as:

The **Beaten Boy**, in memory of a rough childhood;
The **Rebellious Adolescent**, in memory of troubled teenage years;
The **Biker**, in memory of his years with a motorcycle club;
The **Monk**, in memory of his religious conversion; and
The **Hypnotist**, in memory of his present career.

At different times these "parts" of himself might become active and affect his behavior and thoughts. He will seem very different if the "Monk" is active than if the "Biker" part is active. However, these "parts" are simply memories. His personality is the sum of all of these parts, plus other things. We all have such "parts."

Some hypnotists who believe in reincarnation consider their past lives to be "parts" for purposes of this method.

Parts Theories have a long history in hypnotism. Perhaps the best know hypnotist who advocated for this method was Charles Tebbetts. However, there are other systems such as the Inner Voice Dialogue method of Hal Stone, or the Internal Family Systems theory of Richard Schwartz. Our use of the Centrum is simply another form of Parts Theory.

In this implementation of Parts Theory we take a moment in the third step of our Spiritual Hypnotism Method to imagine all of our "parts" using a specific image.

Imagine each part as if it were an ellipse. Then, assemble the ellipses so that they all overlap at one point, like the pedals of a flower. The point where all our parts touch is the Centrum. It represents the most integrated and complete idea of our personality possible.

Imagine yourself moving though the center of this "flower" and proceed to the fourth step of our Spiritual Hypnotism Method.

Then in the fifth step repeat an autosuggestion about the healing of our target person.

As an example: Imagine that I wish to do a healing session for a relative named Tony, who is ill with cancer.

1. First, I induce myself into self-hypnotism using any of a number of favorite techniques. Then the trance is progressively deepened by reflection on the awe and mystery of the universe;
2. Next, I let my imagination run to the possibilities for good that can exist in our universe;
3. I call to mind my "parts" and reflect on who I have been in the past (the Beaten Boy, Rebellious Adolescent, Biker, Monk and Hypnotist), then I imagine these parts coming together and overlapping to create the Centrum. I imagine myself moving through the Centrum.
4. Fourth, I imagine what Tony's life might be like if his cancer is controlled, and finally

5. using the Master's Voice, I say to myself the auto-suggestion "Tony is healthy and well."

We use the Centrum as it has a way of focusing the mind of the hyp-notist in a unique fashion. Weiman and Murphy would both consider this a way of summoning the "higher self" of the hypnotist to attend the hypnotic session.

While theological constructs such as a "higher self" go beyond the scope of our curriculum, the clergy who have created this curriculum do find that this technique adds something special to the hypnotic process.

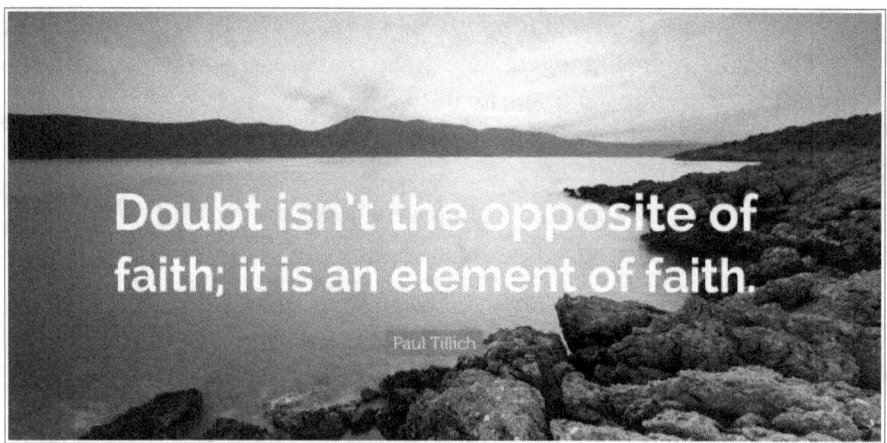

Doubt isn't the opposite of faith; it is an element of faith.

Paul Tillich

Section VI:
Special Dynamics & Considerations

In the following pages are a number of chapters by specialists in their fields of hypnotism. Each piece offers perspective on a particular issue, arena, or dynamic of working with and within spiritual distress.

The first chapter lifts up recent insights in the application of attachment theory to the nature of religion and spirituality. More important than armchair psychology for describing people, this short essay focuses on how the insights of attachment in relationship to a client's spirituality can guide the Spiritual Hypnotism Practitioner in finding resources to be developed in order to help the client build a more secure relationship with their higher power.

We welcome the perspective of Chris Lemig, a transpersonal hypnotist and former Tibetan Buddhist monk, on how Buddhists handle spiritual distress and what techniques and strategies might be particularly beneficial or accessible to clients from a Buddhist religious, philosophical, or cultural background.

President-emeritus of the NGH Clergy Special Interest Group, Rev. Dr. Timothy Jones invites readers to spend a moment clarifying the ethics of working with spiritual distress specifically. It is highly recommended and expected that all Spiritual Hypnotism Practitioners abide by the Code of Ethics and Standards of Practice of the National Guild of Hypnotists, available on the NGH website, www.ngh.net. Jones takes us one informative step further, examining the unique dynamics of spiritually-oriented hypnosis.

Finally, we conclude this section with a brief discussion of ethical meaning-making in suffering. It is tremendously important that we do not minimize or dismiss the genuineness of suffering in our attempts to make a client feel better. It is better to admit the reality of suffering and not apologize for it than to try to justify it or explain it away. Taking a moment to seat that understanding in ourselves will be of profound value to our clients.

Attachment Theory in Spiritual Work
by Christian Skoorsmith, MA, PsyD(c), FNGH

Attachment theory offers a compelling lens through which to examine the qualities of and possibilities within spirituality. Originally developed by John Bowlby and furthered by Mary Ainsworth, attachment theory believes the bonds and interactions between infants and their primary caregivers shape an individual's emotional and social development throughout life. When applied to the context of spirituality and suffering, however, attachment theory provides an additional framework for understanding how early attachment experiences can influence one's religious beliefs, practices, and experiences – offering a vision for how we might encourage healthier, more positive and meaningful spiritual experiences as a result (Pickard & Nelson-Becker, 2011).

Generally, attachment theory identifies a number of different "styles" of attachment: secure, anxious, avoidant, and disorganized (Shaver & Mikulincer, 2012). These styles are formed based on the responsiveness and availability of the caregiver, and they can also be seen reflected in one's conception of divinity or source of meaning. Secure attachment, characterized by trust and a sense of safety, is developed when caregivers are consistently responsive. Anxious attachment arises from inconsistent caregiver responses, leading to uncertainty and anxiety. Avoidant attachment develops when caregivers are emotionally unavailable or rejecting, resulting in a tendency to distance oneself emotionally. Disorganized attachment often stems from abusive or chaotic caregiving environments, leading to confusion and fear. Since its introduction in 1958, attachment theory has been so effective in therapeutic environments, it has been expanded to other disciplines, such as evolutionary theory and religion (Granqvist, 2012).

These attachment styles profoundly influence not only personal relationships but also spiritual experiences and susceptibility to spiritual distress (Ellison et al., 2012; Henderson & Kent, 2022; Zarzycka, 2019). People (individuals and cultures) often conceptualize their relationship with God in ways that mirror their early attachment experiences with caregivers (Granqvist et al., 2020). For instance, individuals with **secure attachment** styles often perceive God as a reliable and loving presence. Their faith tends to be stable and comforting, providing a sense of security and support in times of difficulty. Studies (Rindt-Hoffman et al., 2019) have shown that secure attachment correlates with a positive religious experience and lower levels of spiritual distress. These individuals tend to engage in religious practices that reinforce their sense of community and belonging, further buffering against spiritual distress.

Those with **anxious attachment**, however, may experience a fluctuating sense of closeness to God. Their relationship with a higher power can be characterized by seeking reassurance and validation. They may view God as unpredictable or as a source of conditional love, mirroring their early interactions with caregivers. This can lead to heightened anxiety about their spiritual worthiness and fear of divine abandonment. Anxiously attached individuals might engage in intense religious practices as a way to seek reassurance and validation, but these practices can also exacerbate their anxiety if they perceive themselves as failing to meet religious expectations.

Meanwhile, people who have **avoidant attachment** styles, who have experienced emotional unavailability or rejection from caregivers, often maintain a distant relationship with spirituality. They may view religious practices as irrelevant or find it difficult to engage emotionally with spiritual concepts. This detachment can lead to a sense of spiritual emptiness or disconnect, contributing to existential concern. Avoidantly attached individuals might reject religious beliefs outright or engage in them only superficially, which can prevent them from accessing the potential comfort and community support that religious engagement can provide.

Disorganized attachment results from caregiving that is both frightening and chaotic. These kinds of early experiences often lead to a view of relationships as conflicted and unstable. Unsurprisingly, this attachment style in turn often translates into a turbulent spiritual life. Individuals may oscillate between intense devotion and rejection of spiritual beliefs, experiencing profound spiritual distress and confusion. Their relationship with a Great Other is often characterized by fear, ambivalence, and contradictory feelings. As a result, this chaotic spiritual history can exacerbate feelings of instability and distress in many areas of life, especially regarding spiritual dimensions of experience, making it challenging to find spiritual peace or solace.

The purpose of briefly laying out these styles of "spiritual attachment" is not to armchair psychologize clients or even diagnose an attachment style. (Unless one is licensed to diagnose or perform psychotherapy, generally hypnotists wouldn't engage in those anyway.) This merely introduces another way to conceive of a context for spiritual distress, to recognize what liabilities might be at play and what resources might be available, and to imagine one aspect of helping clients through their journey of spiritual distress.

For instance, we might recognize a potential resource or area of need, depending on what conception of divinity the client presents. Those with securely attached feelings toward their higher power frequently benefit from social engagement in supportive religious practices, rituals, traditions, and observances. Anxiously attached individuals – or those who exhibit that style of relationship with their Great Other – may need more reassurance of unconditional spiritual love and support, before a focus on addressing the particulars of spiritual distress. Clients who harbor an avoidant relationship with the Holy might require gentle, non-threatening encouragement to explore deeper or different spiritual insight or understanding, in order to help them find purposeful, personal meaning. While not unique to them, people exhibiting a disorganized attachment (a deity who is chaotic and frightening, or who has a history of vacillating between extremes in devotion/rejection or in certainty/confusion) often benefit from the intentional creation of a consistent, safe spiritual environment in which to discern, explore, and navigate their conflicted feelings.

One aspect of our work in addressing spiritual distress in our clients should be an attentiveness to **fostering environments and practices that promote security, trust, and positive relational experiences**. We want our work with clients (the therapeutic relationship, our voice and methods, our office or online space) to model acceptance, openness, and positive expectation. Essentially, we want to facilitate movement toward a secure attachment style within the client's own spirituality – while keeping faith with their own spiritual journey, values, and traditions as they see fit. Of course, we do not pass judgment on anyone's beliefs or practices (as long as such objectivity falls within our scope of practices – in many states, hypnotists are mandatory reporters of abuse of children and vulnerable adults, for instance). However, we can offer the client the opportunity to engage in their own spiritual vision with the healthiest understanding possible for them.

There are a number of strategies we can undertake to help individuals develop a secure spiritual attachment. All of these should be considered only insofar as they can be introduced in keeping with the client's own spiritual understanding. First among them is **promoting a loving and accepting view of the divine**. We can emphasize unconditional love and unqualified worth by speaking of the Holy as unconditionally loving and accepting. This helps counteract fears of rejection and fosters a sense of security. Consider using any positive religious imagery and narratives the client brings or can be identified in their religious tradition or spiritual understanding. Remember not to be pollyanish about or dismissive of struggle, pain, suffering, and doubt. One need not negate the genuineness of suffering in order to understand it is (or can be) meaningful and purposeful. Emphasizing the places where the client's own conception of the divine is nurturing and supportive can build resources, resilience, and perspective.

Additionally, to whatever extent is possible and appropriate, **encouraging healthy religious practices** can be beneficial to many clients. Naturally, not all clients will be part of a spiritual or religious community, and some may have (very) negative reactions toward such institutions based on past experiences. So, be judicious in this recommendation. Community and intentional networks of support have been shown to buffer against distress particularly in issues or areas where identity is a factor. While "actual" community can have tremendous benefits, we all know other people can be demanding, and some clients will not be well served under those expectations. However, even individual practices that have a communal element can answer this need, such as meditation at a certain time when others will also be doing the same thing or focusing prayer on some larger or shared concern. Consistency can build a sense of reliability and trust – in community with others and in one's own life, in the community of one's own mind (and all the parts of a person, some of whom might be slower to trust even an individual's best intentions for themselves). Finding rich, ritual, supportive community can reinforce a sense of belonging and security. However clients can find or establish that, all the better.

Leading from these first two, we can make our own practice model a relationship that **provides emotional and spiritual support**. Spiritual Hypnotism Practitioners should consistently offer professional care that is empathetic, non-judgmental, and supportive. Our demeanor, dress, and technique should be approachable and communicate that we are available to listen and provide guidance. Our work should be skilled and informed by continual, credible training that gives us tools which facilitate healthy emotional attachment positioning in spiritual issues.

While the form or formality will differ among clients, our work with them should **encourage self-exploration and personal growth**. Engaging in the HOPE process *with* clients (as opposed to *for* clients) encourages them to explore their spiritual beliefs and practices in a safe and supportive environment. Safety and neutrality allows them to explore how they might have been let down by their beliefs, assumptions, community, traditions, or practices, with no expectation or agenda other than their well-being. The even and hovering attention, and the concept of potential space, offer models to us how to hold just such a nonjudgmental and productive container for our client's wrestling with personally important dynamics. Depending on your process of Spiritual Hypnotism, you might consider how to incorporate practices that encourage self-reflection, such as journaling and reflective prayer, which can help individuals process their experiences and develop a deeper understanding of their spirituality.

It has already been said in this curriculum, but bears repeating in the context of encouraging a client's healthy attachment relations with their higher power, that we should be deliberate and attentive in creating an environment where **doubts and questions are welcomed and addressed openly**. This is essential for individuals to feel safe in their spiritual journey, knowing that they will not be judged for their struggles. No topic important to a client is off limits for discussion. No option is off the table at the outset. We know that feeling accepted and valued is crucial for developing a secure attachment. Without fostering an exclusive dependence on the hypnotist for this kind of support, it is vital that the clinical relationship model an accepting, understanding, and validating relationship for the client to develop in their own interpersonal relationships, intrapersonal dynamics, and spiritual life. The client should feel valued in their own being, without qualification, even in their present distress, doubt, brokenness, and unknowing. Spiritual Hypnotism Practitioners model healthy relational behaviors for clients and others, demonstrating empathy, compassion, and unconditional positive regard. Curiosity should be our watchword: stay curious about what a client is experiencing or expressing, about why. Open-ended questions are our best clinical tool in these moments.

Lastly, we lift up the aspects of the Spiritual Hypnotism process that **integrate healing practices**. Many hypnotists already engage in a multitude of techniques for addressing past wounds and traumas that affect clients' interpersonal relationships and self-image. However, we should look for ways to extend those practices to similar dynamics that affect one's attachment to the divine. It is in keeping with the noblest efforts and articulations of Tillich, Wieman, and Murphy, to see a reflection of one's spirituality in one's relationships with and behavior toward others. Practices of forgiveness and reconciliation are tools which can heal relational wounds and foster a sense of peace and security that translates into spiritual understanding as well. After any significant forgiveness or reconciliation work, it might benefit the client to re-enter a space of spiritual assessment, particularly the Spiritual Goals portion – though from the client's own perspective: have they made progress on the goals they identified? Should the goals be rephrased or changed now, given how the client has changed?

Remember that the purpose of being sensitive to the attachment style of the client's spirituality is to offer insight or clarity on potential needs to be met or resources to be built upon. This is not intended to be diagnostic – in fact, it really isn't about the client at all. This is information the Spiritual Hypnotism Practitioner might use to suggest a direction to the work, if at any time a clear direction is not sensed from the client. Of course, holding a safe and nonjudgmental space means allowing for time where there is no explicit direction, and both client and hypnotist are allowed to be worthy enough without the qualification of "something to do."

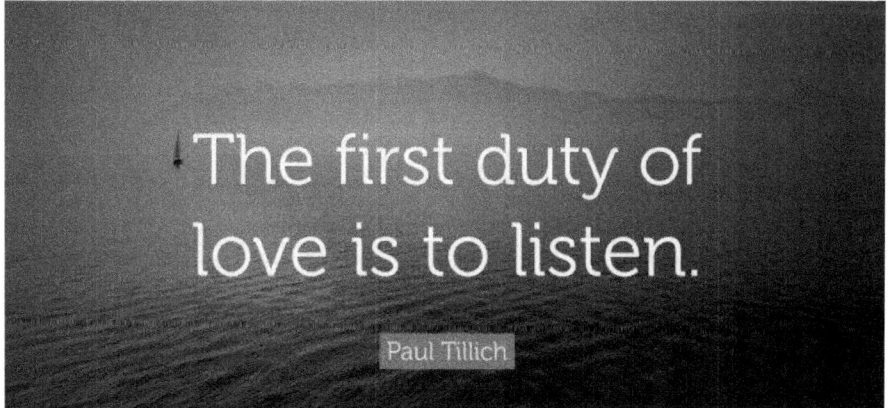

The first duty of love is to listen.

Paul Tillich

References

Ellison, C. G., Bradshaw, M., Kuyel, N., & Marcum, J. P. (2012). Attachment to God, stressful life events, and changes in psychological distress. *Review of Religious Research*, *53*(4), 493-511.

Granqvist, P. (2012). Introduction to the special issue: Advancements in the study of attachment and religion/spirituality. *International Journal for the Psychology of Religion*, *22*(3), 173-179.

Granqvist, P., Mikulincer, M., & Shaver, P. R. (2020). An attachment theory perspective on religion and spirituality. In *The science of Religion, Spirituality, and Existentialism* (pp. 175-186). Academic Press.

Henderson, W. M., & Kent, B. V. (2022). Attachment to God and psychological distress: Evidence of a curvilinear relationship. *Journal for the Scientific Study of Religion*, *61*(1), 161-177.

Pickard, J. G., & Nelson-Becker, H. (2011). Attachment and spiritual coping: Theory and practice with older adults. *Journal of Spirituality in Mental Health*, *13*(2), 138-155.

Rindt-Hoffman, S., Kernes, J. L., & Bui, N. H. (2019). Attachment style, spirituality, and compassionate love among mental health professionals. *Journal of Mental Health Counseling*, *41*(2), 112-126.

Shaver, P. R., & Mikulincer, M. (2012). Attachment theory. In P. A. M. Van Lange, A. W. Kruglanski, & E. T. Higgins (Eds.), *Handbook of theories of psychology* (Vol. 2), pp 160-179. Sage Publications Ltd.

Zarzycka, B. (2019). Parental attachment styles and religious and spiritual struggle: A mediating effect of God image. *Journal of Family Issues*, *40*(5), 575-593.

Integrating Buddhist Philosophy Into Hypnosis Practice: A Guide for Professional Hypnotists
By Chris Lemig, CHT

For professional hypnotists, understanding and respecting the beliefs and worldviews of clients is essential for effectively meeting their needs and helping them achieve their goals. For hypnotists working with Buddhist clients, it is particularly important to grasp the fundamental tenets of Buddhism and tailor our hypnotic approaches towards building rapport and connection. This chapter aims to provide insights into Buddhist beliefs, perspectives on how Buddhists view and deal with life challenges, as well as recommendations for incorporating Buddhist principles into an effective hypnosis session or series of sessions.

Understanding Buddhist Beliefs

Buddhism is a spiritual tradition originating from the teachings of Siddhartha Gautama (the Buddha) that encompasses a diverse array of beliefs, practices, and cultural perspectives. However, several core principles are common to most Buddhist philosophical traditions:

1. The Four Noble Truths
The Four Noble Truths form the foundation of Buddhism and they are considered to be the Buddha's first formal teaching. They outline the reality of suffering, the cause of suffering, the cessation of suffering, and Nirvana, the path to liberation from suffering.

In the First Noble Truth, the Buddha observes that human existence is characterized by *dukkha*. This Sanskrit term has usually been translated as "suffering" but a better interpretation may be "unsatisfactoriness." It's not just the gross sufferings of pain, disappointment, and loss that make human life problematic. Even relatively pleasant experiences such as worldly success, sensory enjoyment, and good health are subject to impermanence and decay. Because nothing ultimately lasts, we are left feeling dissatisfied no matter how much happiness we may experience over the course of a lifetime.

The Second Noble Truth explains that this experience of suffering or unsatisfactoriness is caused by our deeply ingrained habit of clinging and grasping at external experiences. This habit is rooted in our fundamental ignorance about the reality of how things actually exist. Not fully understanding and accepting that all external phenomena are impermanent, fleeting, and interconnected, we try to hold onto them as if they were independently existing object-experiences and attempt to make them last. This ultimately leads to frustration and is the root cause of human suffering.

Although some people could perceive Buddhism to be a pessimistic philosophy, the Third Noble Truth demonstrates that just the opposite is true. Having established the problem (suffering and unsatisfactoriness) and the cause of the problem (grasping and clinging), the Buddha makes his fundamental assertion: *there is an end to suffering*. The end or cessation of suffering comes about as soon as we fully and deeply understand the impermanent, interdependent nature of phenomena and let go of our entrenched habit of grasping.

Because this is not an easy task, in the Fourth Noble Truth, the Buddha outlines an ethical, spiritual, and philosophical path for bringing about the cessation of suffering. Ethical behavior based on the principle of non-harm mitigates many of life's most egregious forms of suffering. Meditation helps subdue the grasping mind, while practical contemplations on the impermanence and interdependence of all experienceable phenomena lead to a deep sense of spiritual freedom and peace known as "enlightenment" or Nirvana.

2. Impermanence

Buddhist thought highlights the transient nature of all phenomena, emphasizing that nothing is permanent or fixed. While this may seem obvious, most human behavior is deeply influenced by the apparent denial of this basic fact.

Most of us operate under the presumption that things are going to last from moment to moment. We make plans and decisions assuming we're going to live well into old age. We hold onto grudges and resentments for years and decades, long after the original offense took place. We defend and impose–sometimes even violently–beliefs, ideas, and values that inevitably change over time.

All of these types of attitudes and behaviors point to the deep resistance we have toward the truth of impermanence. Out of our longing for certainty and familiarity, we desperately want things to last. Most Buddhists are no different from anyone else in this regard. Nonetheless, it can be helpful to offer gentle and compassionate reminders of the reality of an ever-changing world when guiding your clients through major transitions, grief, loss, and crisis.

3. Emptiness

Central to Buddhist thought is the concept of emptiness, which maintains that there is no independently existing essence to any phenomena. This includes human beings.

Whenever you attempt to isolate the distinctness, or independent existence, of any person or thing, you quickly find it can be broken down into an infinite array of interrelated factors, parts, causes, and conditions that are continuously changing.

In reality, there are actually no concrete, independently existing "things" anywhere. Rather, everything we can observe is a continuously unfolding, interrelated process. In fact, all phenomena we can perceive are so interconnected through a vast web of causality that the Universe can ultimately only be understood as a single, vastly complex singularity.

Complex philosophy aside, the concept of emptiness reveals that rather than being separate and alone, we are all deeply interconnected with everyone and everything around us. This can be a powerful and comforting reframe when dealing with someone familiar with Buddhist ideas who is navigating a period of spiritual distress.

4. Compassion and Loving-Kindness

An essential part of the Buddhist path is cultivating compassion and loving-kindness towards oneself and others. Not only do love and compassion offer a counterbalance to the often heady philosophical aspects of Buddhism, but they are in themselves antidotes to the hurts and sufferings of human life. In fact, a Buddhist definition of compassion is the wish that ourselves and others be free of suffering and its causes.

As part of the mental, emotional, and spiritual training for cultivating the mind of compassion, Buddhists will contemplate the fact that all beings want nothing less than freedom from suffering that results in a state of ultimate happiness. Realizing this fully can be a lifetime learning process. However, as we train in empathy, compassion, and loving-kindness, we can begin to experience a softening of our own hearts, finding it easier to be more patient and loving towards ourselves and others.

Whether or not your Buddhist client has a strong compassion practice or not, reminding them of the power of love and compassion–especially towards themselves–can be a powerful aid in moving the session towards its ultimate aim: the alleviation of suffering.

It's important to recognize that Buddhist practitioners will have varying degrees of understanding of these core tenets and beliefs. Some people may simply feel they align with Buddhist teachings and ideas but lack any formal training or practice. Others may have extensive experience with rituals and prayers but have less interest in applying the essence of these practices in daily life. Whatever the case, many people who identify as Buddhist will likely have some familiarity with the above topics. The degree of familiarity, understanding, and level of practice can be clarified during the initial Spiritual Assessment.

How Buddhists View and Deal with Life Challenges

Buddhism offers a profound perspective on addressing life's challenges, viewing them as opportunities for growth, learning, and spiritual development. Much of modern society treats our pain and discomfort by only addressing the symptoms. Distraction through entertainment, pharmaceutical pain suppression, and other superficial approaches are like bandaids that only offer temporary relief. Rather than resisting or denying difficulties, sincere Buddhists seek to understand the root causes of suffering in order to find a more permanent solution. Through the trainings of mindfulness, compassion, and wisdom Buddhists aim to address those root causes in a more meaningful way.

Key approaches in Buddhist practice include:

1. Mindfulness Meditation

Buddhists employ mindfulness practices to develop present-moment awareness, allowing them to observe thoughts, emotions, and sensations without attachment or aversion. This makes Buddhist clients uniquely positioned to be successful hypnosis patients.

One of the main reasons we experience intense states of emotional suffering, like anxiety, fear, disappointment, and so on, is that we are immersed in the feeling. Essentially, we are identified with the problem state to such a degree that we fail to recognize that it is a temporary experience and not the essence of who we are.

A mindfulness practitioner, whether they are Buddist or not, will have some ability to step back and observe whatever feelings or emotions that are coming up during the period of spiritual distress. This is actually similar to the common hypnotic strategy of "dual awareness" whereby one can experience a painful memory or feeling without becoming fully associated with it. In doing so, it becomes easier to see the problem state from different perspectives, reframe it in different contexts, and become open to new learning and solutions that might otherwise go unnoticed.

During the Spiritual Assessment, ask your client what their experience is with mindfulness meditation. You can also explain the similarities of hypnosis and meditation as both being states of inner focus and awareness. Then, you can collaborate with your client to find ways to leverage their mindfulness training as a resource for change and growth.

2. Acceptance of Impermanence

As we've seen, resistance to the truth of impermanence is both a direct cause of suffering as well as a contributing factor to intensifying it. When we experience a painful loss or undesired change in our life's plan, many of us fall prey to the habit of dwelling on the negative experience. We may feel "singled out" by the universe or that some malevolent force is punishing us for some mysterious (and likely unjust) reason. We forget that change in and of itself is neutral. It's only our conditioned beliefs, attitudes, and judgments that color this neutrality with definitions of "good" and "bad".

By more fully recognizing the impermanent nature of things, it becomes easier to accept the natural ebb and flow of life's inevitable changes. Even experiences as profoundly life-changing as death, terminal illness, and

catastrophic loss can be seen as universal occurrences that every human being will eventually face in some form or another. Without denying deep
emotions of grief and sadness, we can, as Buddhist teacher Pema Chodron
advises, "lean into" the suffering. In this way, we avoid the danger of simply
bypassing or avoiding our pain, instead seizing an opportunity to find
deeper meaning in it.

This doesn't mean that all Buddhists will have a perfect understanding and acceptance of the truth of impermanence. Recognizing the impermanent nature of all things is an ongoing and lifelong practice. However,
most Buddhists will be familiar, if not comfortable, with the idea that everything will eventually pass. One should still be mindful and compassionate
when helping a client reframe spiritually distressing change as impermanent. But in the right setting and context, it can help bring about a deeply
healing perspective shift.

3. Compassionate Action and Attitude

Like many spiritual traditions, Buddhists are encouraged to engage
in acts of compassion and altruism, seeking to alleviate the suffering of others and contribute positively to the world. However, this need not be only in
the form of physical actions.

Although acts of charity and service are beneficial, the main point is
that we cultivate and strengthen a more natural tendency to think of others,
at least as much as we normally think of ourselves and our own interests. In
fact, Buddhists are taught to carefully examine their secret motivations *before* engaging in compassionate action. Are we being generous so we can get
something in return? Do we engage in philanthropy seeking acknowledg-
ment and praise? Is our volunteer work a means to prove to ourselves or
others that we are "good" people?

These often unconscious motivations are rooted in the grasping and
mis-identification of a permanently existing self that the Buddha pointed to
as the cause of our suffering in the Second Noble Truth.

Self-awareness of these hidden motivations and desires gives us the
opportunity to face our "shadow" parts of self-centeredness and grasping.
When we recognize and take ownership of these parts, we can actively begin to free ourselves from the unnecessary suffering they cause. There are
many Buddhist meditation practices that focus on generating loving, empathetic, and compassionate thoughts and emotions. These practices have the

potential to transform long-standing habits of self-centeredness and, over time, naturally result in more compassionate thoughts and feelings toward others.

4. Cultivation of Wisdom

Through contemplation and insight practices, Buddhists develop wisdom into the true nature of reality, transcending conventional perceptions of time-bound permanence and attaining a deeper understanding of who and what we are.

One powerful contemplation follows a line of inquiry into our true nature and identity. Most of us take for granted the notion of an independently existing and continuous self or "I". In this practice, a Buddhist will challenge this assumption and begin an earnest inward search for this concrete self. Where does it exist? Am "I" my body, my mind, my brain, my emotions? Am "I" any of the many labels and concepts I and others identify as "me"? Am "I" the totality of all of my memories, learning, and experiences?

Through this practice, one quickly discovers that the sense of "I" is actually quite elusive and cannot be pointed to directly and definitively. The reality is that we do not exist as a static "thing" but as a dynamic and ever-changing process unfolding in consciousness and awareness. This deeper wisdom and insight into our true nature has the natural effect of liberating us from the suffering caused by grasping at the illusion of an independently existing self.

Suggestions for Hypnosis Sessions

Incorporating some of your client's values and beliefs into your hypnosis sessions is an important part of developing connection and rapport. When you make the attempt to "speak the language" of your client, you build a bridge of trust that reduces resistance to open communication and change. The following suggestions for how to work with Buddhist hypnosis clients can help improve the quality of both the sessions themselves and the outcomes your client experiences post-session.

1. Cultivate Mindful Presence and Positive Motivation

Begin each session by cultivating a mindful presence, inviting both yourself and your client to anchor in the present moment. Encourage slow, conscious breathing and awareness of bodily sensations to establish a foundation of mindfulness. Auditory sensations, such as the sounds inside or outside the room, as well as the sound of your voice, can be reframed as focal points of alert attention and interest rather than distraction. In fact, any sensory experience can be utilized as an object of mindful awareness. Bring your own awareness of what you observe in the environment, your client's body, and even yourself to creatively find ways to foster mindfulness.

Once grounded in the present moment, encourage the client to formulate a positive motivation for the session. This can be a simple aspiration such as, "May all the work we do here today be of the highest possible benefit to ourselves and all beings." Invite your client to allow their subconscious mind to play with this motivation. What would the highest possible benefit look and feel like? What new learnings and discoveries are going to be made by the subconscious mind during the session and how are they going to result in more wisdom, insight, love, and compassion?

2. Frame Challenges as Opportunities for Growth

When discussing life challenges, reframe them as opportunities for growth and self-discovery. Emphasize the transient nature of difficulties and the potential for transformation through compassionate self-reflection and acceptance. It can also be pointed out that the challenges we face give us a deeper insight into human suffering in general, allowing us to be more empathetic, patient, and kind towards others.

For example, the end of a long term relationship can be viewed as an opportunity to celebrate that the client has demonstrated the capacity to stay committed to another person amidst all the challenges they faced together. The end of a relationship can also be seen as a way to cultivate empathy and compassion for other human beings who have undergone and will undergo similar losses and upheavals.

3. Use Metaphors and Symbolism

Incorporate metaphors and symbolic language that resonate with Buddhist teachings. A classic image is a lotus flower emerging from muddy waters to symbolize enlightenment arising from suffering and adversity. Utilize imagery that evokes themes of impermanence, interconnectedness, and liberation. The planting, sprouting, and harvesting of vegetables through the seasons. The snake shedding its skin or the life cycle of egg to caterpillar to chrysalis to butterfly are powerful images of change, growth, and being "reborn" anew.

Focus the client's attention on the harmony and interconnectedness of all the organs in their body, working in concert to support all life's processes. Tell a story of a person such as Nelson Mandela, wrongly imprisoned, who is released into freedom, ultimately enriched by the ordeal, and able to bring a boon of wisdom, love, and compassion to the world.

Another powerful metaphor that is effective for quieting the mind is to imagine all thoughts and feelings floating by like leaves on a stream. For clients who find it difficult to focus, invoke the image of inner and outer sensory experiences being like waves cresting momentarily on the surface of a deep ocean of awareness.

4. Integrate Loving-Kindness Meditation

Guide clients through loving-kindness meditations to cultivate compassion towards oneself and others.

A basic loving-kindness practice begins with generating feelings of love for oneself. Encourage the repetition of phrases such as "May I be happy, may I be healthy, may I be safe, may I live with ease."

For many people, this may actually be quite challenging as the idea of "self-love" is often fraught with feelings of unworthiness, shame, and low self-esteem. If this is the case, either help your client begin to work through that resistance or set it aside for the time being.

Next, suggest that your client bring up an image of a person they unconditionally love and care for. This could be a child, a partner, a close friend, or a family member. Invite them to bring up and intensify warm-hearted feelings for this person, imagining them experiencing more and more happiness, joy, and well-being.

At this point, it can be helpful for your client to visualize, imagine, or simply sense a white light in their heart. This light is filled with all the love, kindness, and compassion they feel for their loved one. Suggest that they imagine rays of this light radiate out into the world, touching the hearts of more and more people as the light reaches out across the whole globe.

This visualization can be accompanied by an aspiration similar to the one above, such as, "May all beings be happy. May all beings be healthy, safe, and live at ease."

For the client struggling with self love, you can end this meditation with this powerful resource state of love and kindness being directed towards themselves.

5. Foster Equanimity and Acceptance

Encourage clients to develop equanimity and acceptance towards life's ups and downs. This can be done skillfully and compassionately by guiding them to recognizing the futility of clinging to fixed outcomes and the liberating power of embracing impermanence with equanimity.

The reality is that all things change whether or not we accept this fact. Resistance only adds unnecessary pain and suffering to the situation. When we can accept change–even difficult and unwanted change–we become open to the possibility of learning from that change. In fact, it is only because of change that we are able to learn anything at all. If we lived in a permanent and unchanging world, then no new experiences would be possible.

Equanimity is ultimately a state of freedom, love, and joy rather than cold aloofness and insensitivity. Through equanimity we are able to more clearly see the natural, miraculous, and wondrous displays of creation all around us. When we allow things to be as they are, without grasping at them in an attempt to make them last or fit into our limited set of beliefs and expectations, we become free to enjoy the ever-unfolding dance of appearances.

Conclusion

Integrating these principles and suggestions into our hypnosis practice can enhance the support we offer Buddhist clients on their journey to the other side of spiritual distress. But it's not just Buddhists who can benefit from these ideas and practices. As in many spiritual traditions, Buddhism transmits universal truths and wisdom. Mindful self-awareness, acceptance of impermanence, and the cultivation of a more loving and compassionate heart can be useful resources for anyone experiencing periods of difficulty, regardless of their religious associations. Buddhist philosophy and principles like mindfulness, compassion, and wisdom, when combined with hypnosis, can serve as powerful tools for transformation, healing, and spiritual growth.

The Ethics of Dealing with Spiritual Distress
By Rev. Timothy Jones, B.Min, MA, PhD(c), FNGH, OB

What is spiritual distress?

First, one must ask, what is spirituality, and how does a disruption occur?

In life, regardless of cultural indoctrination or societal norms, humans develop beliefs about what is important to them, like how to act in certain situations, or how to reflect on different circumstances, or how to elicit behavioral response from others.

Those beliefs then develop into life values and become inherently present, for example being polite vs. gruff as a manner of being.

Those life experiences involve an intertwinement of meaning and purpose along with hopes of a positive (or negative) expectation and an awareness of a connection (or not) beyond the material world.

For the disenfranchised religious, it could be they were traumatized by their religious body when told they'll be separated from God, face social ruin or go to hell if they don't adhere to specific traditions or beliefs; or, if they embraced alternative beliefs, and upon transgression that they'd be denied a place in an afterlife.

We've found though that people who lose faith in a particular religious philosophy or religious denomination still hold out hope of a Universal Power, or God, and are comforted by that spiritual belief in times of trouble.

For the non-practicing religious, spirituality involves having faith and trust in a higher power, a transcendent force or being supporting a deeper spiritual reality than the one provided for them by the traditional religiosity they've experienced in some way or another.

That sense of spirituality can provide comfort, strength, and guidance in difficult times and can be a source of inspiration, motivation, and inner peace.

And the atheist, for example the soldier exposed to kill-or-be-killed situations contradicting their upbringing, jettisons all beliefs of a God once active in the taking of lives.

The author has chaplained several Canadian Special Forces members who, when asked specifics about their faith, answered that, in situations where there seemed no way out, they asked "whoever" for help in the moment, but were careful to couch that with the belief that *"there's no God on the battlefield."*

Spiritual distress, then, is a disruption of a person's belief system when they question a source they once turned to for hope, love, comfort, guidance or protection.

The distressed begin to doubt their long-held beliefs about God, or their higher power, or wherever they found meaning, and when they can't sense this guiding meaning anymore, it can affect their entire being – physically, mentally and spiritually.

Diagnosing Distress

How does one determine that a client is spiritually distressed?

The signs of Spiritual Distress are usually when one exhibits behaviors of sadness, anger, despair, or anxiety. According to the findings of a recent study (Eshghi, 2023, p. 2839), "lack of peace, hopelessness, anger, change in the meaning given to life, fear, and crying were the most defining features in the reviewed texts for the diagnosis of spiritual distress."

They overtly question people and institutions with whom they were formerly in agreement, such as clergy, practitioners, institutions or helping entities.

You'll hear them question the meaning of their suffering, asking *"Why now?"* and *"Why me?"* along with expressions of feelings of emptiness, a loss of life direction and feelings of abandonment.

Those in spiritual distress may also ask *"Why is this happening to me?"*, *"Why has God let this happen?"*, *"What's my purpose now?"*, *"This is not fair"*, *"I'm scared"* and *"I don't know how I'm going to cope."*

You'll notice these expressions of life frustration are very similar to those of people starting to consider ending their lives.

Examples

There will be fuller explanations in this book but as a Minister, the causes I've run across are family members shocked upon the death of an elderly but very healthy family member.

Similarly, the unexpected death of a pre-natal or peri-natal child, of a pre-pubescent child, of a teenager or young adult all raise unending questions as to why.

Unfortunately, lack of distinct and conforming church policy can also shatter a family's beliefs. For example, I took on counseling almost a whole family of, to that point, devout Catholic family when the presiding priest at Grandfather's funeral intoned that we should pray for "John" as he isn't able to pray where he is.

As a friend of the family, they came to me, in anguish and confusion, asking if their loved grandfather was in hell? Where was he? Was he a supersized sinner in the eyes of the church? Why could he not pray in heaven?

The Catholic Church does NOT teach that the dead cannot pray for their living family, or to the Holy Father – unless they are indeed in purgatory. And even the Holy See has officially said that hell is perhaps a place but that all souls go to the Father.

What some clergy incorrectly (in my humble opinion) postulate though is that all people should make themselves right with God before they transition, for they will not be able to afterwards.

That philosophy is viewed as a continuing device to control man both by churches and by the rabid evangelicals who use scare tactics along with fear to make congregations adhere.

We've even heard pastors in service profess that all souls go to hell for a time before God calls them up. *("I'm going where?")*

Indeed, although metaphysicians and other spirit-aware humans agree there are people in 'the dark' as a result of life choices and influences, as hypnotists, we can help bring them to the light with the help of angels.

Regardless of how negative human beliefs were propagated, they are a state of mind that we, as counselors, can help mitigate.

Ethical Issues

There could be quite a few ethical issues a counselor might confront but the primary one is that of trying to impose, influence or convert the client to the practitioner's own faith or belief set.

It is that very roadblock that pastors, priests, imams, rabbis, chaplains and spiritual counselors face in society in general as those rejecting a higher power think the theologically trained will try convert them "back to the path."

At the same time, it is certainly appropriate for all counselors to gauge the client's beliefs and how importantly they play in their life during the intake, but the clinician should approach the issue(s) without crossing a religious ethical boundary.

Some of the risks when incorporating religion and spirituality in counseling are the imposition of values, discrimination(s) no matter how unintentional, ineffective or singularly meaning communication, lack of sensitivity, or being too focused on the religion and spirituality aspect rather than addressing the perhaps underlying reason the client came to you.

Don't get it wrong though. By mutual agreement, a therapist can encourage a client to utilize their faith as a coping skill. This has been effectively used to treat everything from anxiety to substance abuse.

However, if the particular brand of religion or spirituality is not one the clinician is experienced with, or feels they can not remain unbiased about, since they've already come to you, consider offering the client a hypnotherapeutic session centered around Ego Enhancement to bolster them, and refer out.[1]

The biggest concern about incorporating religion and spirituality in sessions is when there is a difference in religion or spirituality between the helping professional and the client.

Even in cases where both the counselor and the client have the same professed religion, there might still be some major difference in values between the two – as in the dead cannot pray example we quoted.

In such cases, whose religious viewpoint(s) are to be followed?

---

1   *One side note, a clinician needs to be careful in regards to religion/spirituality and certain disorders such as bi-polar and schizophrenia, where beliefs and practice can be more harmful than helpful when the client is suffering from these disorders.*

There are coaches, instructors and teachers who see religion and spirituality as an important part of counseling which have proven to be effective.

However, in their rush to fame and fortune, some trainers trying to develop a following insist their wording be used in every session with every client verbatim.

Do not do that. Reject those teachers. Every client and their perspective is different. Good training is presented as general guidelines, not carved-in-stone verbiage.

Just like any other tools, those approaches can either be beneficial when properly utilized, or bring more harm than good if abused, whether purposefully or not.

Be warned also that the traditional medical models we sometimes have to battle against may pathologize challenging emotional reactions as manifestations of mental illness.

Spiritual Distress especially is viewed by the medical community as the SOP to "call the chaplain," but again, if not trained in the area, and suicidality, REFER OUT.

You don't need the session fee that badly and there's always a trained practitioner nearby.

RECOMMENDATION – An excellent 2-day, intensive, interactive and practice-dominated *Applied Suicide Intervention Skills Training Course (ASIST)* is taught worldwide to military, schools, nurses and the civil population by LIVING WORKS.

Your Approach

Understand that your client is the expert on themselves. They will tell you everything you need to know to work with them ... if you listen. The way they dress, talk or express themselves may have absolutely nothing to do with what they're trying to tell you.

The key is to LISTEN WITH A "BEGINNERS MIND" – The idea behind this strategy is that you take all of the things you know — all of your brilliant opinions, all of your reason and logic, even your cherished beliefs, and you put it all on the shelf for awhile. (it'll still be there when you get back!)

A "beginner's mind" is a practice rooted in Zen. It is the mind innocent of any preconceptions, expectations, judgments and prejudices. The beginner's mind is just present to explore and observe and see "things as-they-are."

Unfortunately, once you develop the belief that you've "heard all this before" *(and you probably have)*, you've closed your mind and are comparing what you're hearing to what you already do or do not believe.

You are then prejudicially either agreeing or disagreeing with your client in your mind as to what is being said. Again, first rule, it is not what YOU believe, it's what the client believes. And who knows, maybe they're telling the truth. No matter, at the time it's spoken to you, it is THEIR truth.

So, if you listen with a beginners mind, you'll learn something new about something already known from every session, and in realizing how much you don't know, you'll become the insightful person who takes delight in each new client, to the client's benefit.

Benefits of Spiritual Well-Being

The spiritually healthy have an increased ability to find meaning in the midst of illness, injury and trauma.

They have an increased ability to accept lived experience by rejecting negativity and embracing positivity.

During illness, they have an increased ability to cope with pain, nausea and discomfort for an improved sense of well-being and are motivated to complete the tasks of healing, both mentally and physically.

They exhibit noticeably decreased feelings of anxiety, depression, anger and loneliness than when struggling with spiritual conflict.

They also experience decreased alcohol and drug involvement and/or abuse and are noticeably more content in their lives.

Your Takeaway

Consider this, you don't have to proselytize, quote, advise or counsel, all you have to do to give your client a healing session is to project a positive, non-judgmental presence for them to recognize.

If you have faith, they will pick that up from you.

If you are secure and at peace with yourself, your client will pick that up off you.

If you are caring and understanding, they will pick that up off you, too.

Sometimes, just being reminded of what they used to feel themselves when spiritually balanced is enough to start them on the healing path.

Feel free to lead the way.

Blessings.

Namaste

References

Eshghi, F., Nikfarid, L., & Zareiyan, A. (2023). An integrative review of defining characteristic of the nursing diagnosis "spiritual distress". *Nursing Open*, *10*(5), 2831-2841. https://doi.org/10.1002/nop2.1574

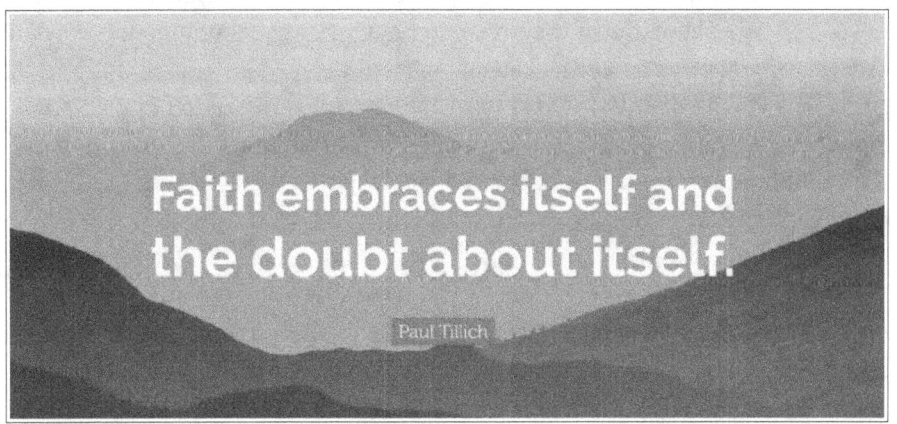

Faith embraces itself and the doubt about itself.

Paul Tillich

Job and Smallpox:
Lessons for Ethical Meaning–Making
Out of Suffering

By Christian Skoorsmith, MA, PsyD(c), FNGH

"For we were born only yesterday and know nothing,
and our days on earth are but a shadow."
Job 8:9

The story of Job often holds an outsized place in the minds of bibli-cally-minded people who are struggling with suffering – their own or that of a loved one. Almost as if it speaks directly to our fears and answers us with the sweet balm of encouragement, purpose, and confidence. The story of Job – dramatic and graphic as it is at points – tells us that suffering is not final, that injustice will not ultimately stand, that there is an Intelligence and Pur-pose in the mechanisms of the universe beyond our reckoning, that we can rely on the universe to be, in the end, fair and good. Who wouldn't find that good news in the midst of trial and tribulation? A recent popular study guide read: "The Book of Job is, in the end, a morality tale designed to show that people must trust in God, even in the face of adversity, because every-thing happens for a purpose." Except....

That it is a gross misreading of the story, historically and textually inaccurate, and a disservice to the genuineness of suffering humans experi-ence. I do not wish to remove anyone's crutch, believe me. At the same time, I am wary of how crutches have been wielded as weapons (consciously and unconsciously) that harm rather than heal. They would deny an uncomfort-able truth for the short-term benefit of the patina of peace. There is an ethi-cal issue at stake here for people who would be guiding the meaning-mak-ing of others in difficult circumstances.

Whether or not the Bible is authoritative for you personally, you will almost certainly come into contact with someone for whom it is. Regardless, the story of Job offers an important object lesson about ethical meaning-making in the face of unnecessary suffering. Allow me to spin a yarn for a moment.

For those unfamiliar with the story, Job is a "blameless," God-fearing man – which is important for the plot-line. (Only two people in the Bible are said to have never sinned: Jesus and Job.) For some reason (reasons differ, depending on the version or revision one reads), Job experiences a series of tragedies: first losing all his property, then his wife and children suffer and die, and then he suffers extraordinary physical agony himself. His friends and authorities argue why this must be happening to Job – did he sin, did he lose faith, should he repent? What did he do to deserve such punishment? All the while, Job professes both his innocence and his faith (which are essential for the point of the story – if he really *had* sinned, even unknowingly, then there would be no plot). He never "blames" or curses God, despite all the suffering. "Though God slay me, yet will I hope in God" (13:15), and "God knows the way that I take; when God has tested me, I will come forth as gold," Job says, confidently (23:10). Job endures until the end, when God restores him to health, replaces his property, and provides a new wife and children – twice as much and as many as before... as if that makes everything alright, even-steven, no harm no foul. (Obviously, the story was not written from the perspective of his first wife and kids!)

But then, right at the end, Job asks God *Why?* And this is where things get *really* uncomfortable.

You see, in ancient Southwest Asia, this motif was fairly common. It circulated in varied versions among most of the civilizations and cultures of the region. Some noble, undeserving figure would suffer extraordinary and unjust things, in the end being restored and blessed, with the natural justice of the universe affirmed. Suffering, these stories told their audiences, only *seems* like suffering, or only *appears* to be unjust – really, on the whole, the universe is fair... we just cannot see it from our limited viewpoint sometimes. Take heart; stay the course. Rich rewards await those who endure difficulties, exploitation, injustice, and privation. Everything is the way it was meant to be: everything has a purpose. So, really, what you are experiencing isn't 'bad' at all. (Or, certainly not as 'bad' as it appears to us in our provincial perspective.) You see? Doesn't that make you feel better? (Again, cold comfort for Job's wife, kids, and livestock.)

Every *other* version of the story ends this same sort of way: things are put right so everything is good. No worries, people! Suffering isn't *really* suffering, if seen from a larger perspective. It is just a brief episode on the path to paradise. Just look at it differently!

But the story of Job has a twist. Job gets to do what we all want to do: ask God *Why*? *How* is that fair? ("I really liked my first wife, God, and was kinda sweet on some of those kids. Sure, the new ones are great and all, but did the first lot really have to suffer and die?") And, surprisingly, the authors of the biblical story have God answer. And the whole story turns on its head as a result.

God responds with offense: "Where were you when I laid the foundation of the earth? Tell me, if you have understanding. Who determined its measurements – surely you know!" (38:4-5). In other words: Who are you to question me? You know nothing! How dare you question the meaning of the universe – you presume the universe *has* meaning! God mocks Job: "On what were the earth's bases sunk, or who laid the cornerstone?"

The easy interpretation here is that Job just doesn't see the moral arc of the universe the way God does – *that's* why Job doesn't understand. Job's job (and thus ours by moral proxy) is to remain faithful, even in the face of suffering. God ultimately has our back. That's the easy interpretation.

There is this little snag in the narrative, however. After God spends four chapters excoriating Job for his presumption to question the course of the universe, God turns to Job's friends who all the while had been making the case (in various ways) that what was happening to Job ought to make some kind of sense. They were, in their own way, defending God, saying God had to be fair, so Job must deserve it somehow or maybe it isn't all that bad. God lays into them, saying that *Job* was correct this whole time (Job was saying that he did not deserve the suffering, that what was happening was *not* right). His friends were flat wrong: "you have not spoken of me what is right, as my servant Job has done" (42:8).

So – and lean in on this with me – Job was correct that whole time, saying that the suffering and misfortune didn't make sense, and his friends (who were trying to make sense of the suffering) were wrong.

Job comes out the hero, of course (he suffered, after all) – but not because he denied the suffering. His friends wanted to explain the evil away, deny it, say it wasn't really evil (it just appeared to be), the universe is a fair place, God is a just god, blah-blah-blah. But Job said: "No, this does not make sense. It is not right. This is horrible." In the end, Job is vindicated.

This is deeply disorientating. It makes the biblical version of this story virtually unique in ancient West Asian literature. The story goes along just as everyone would expect and then, in the end, it refuses to paint a pretty picture, refuses to say that what happened was OK, was fair, was just. God admits as much by raising Job and rebuking his friends. The book of Job – if we read it all the way to the end – implies that the universe does not 'make sense,' is essentially amoral, is not fair.

The book of Job, then, becomes a long commentary on human psychology and our *desire* for the world to make sense – our predisposition to assume a fairness to the world. We respond to fortune and misfortune as if it were the natural consequence of something we have done or some part of a greater divine plan.

This tendency to invest a sense of fairness into reality might be rooted in early childhood experiences, when we are raised in families, relationships, and cultures that are constructed (more or less) around the idea of natural consequences, justice, just desserts, crime and punishment, and all that. The reason we get angry at cheaters prospering is because we feel like they *shouldn't*. Conservative religious figures will blame hurricanes on the moral failure of the affected regions. We see migrant farmers toiling away in the sun and unreflectively assume that they made poor decisions in their lives and we deserve the fortunate situation we are in. And so on. Humans naturally have a sense of fairness built into us. (Not just humans. Other primates exhibit a native sense of fairness. Even my cats know when one of them gets fed and not the others. They will whine follow me until justice is done.)

However, if we really come to terms with it, the world *is* amoral. Tragedies befall the good and the bad. Fortune crowns those who deserve it and those who do not. We like to tell the story differently, but the success of Bill Gates, Jeff Bezos, Elon Musk, and Paul Allen has just as much to do with chance as with any intention or hard work on their part. The world is nonsensical. We do not often recognize that this is the world we inhabit, but that is the influence of our minds and expectations, not the natural order of the cosmos.

Most of the time, meaningfulness and purpose and justice and fairness are the unspoken principles of the vast majority of our lived experience. (Take traffic laws, for example. We follow the rules so passively that we live as though the rules exist independently of us. Every day. And we *want* everyone to believe that those rules are not up to individual abrogation! Rules don't work if they're optional.)

Only on rare occasions are we thrust into an undeniable recognition of the essential senselessness of the universe. Tragedy, suffering, facing death – our own or that of a loved one – and so on. These experiences bring us face-to-face with the disturbing realization that the cosmos is not friendly, not purposeful, not intelligent or fair. It isn't necessarily *against* us, either. The universe doesn't care. Caring (or not-caring) is a fiction peculiar to our minds. When this foundation to how we live and breathe and move in the world is shown to be sand, that we have built our castles in the clouds, a great deal in us that seemed firm comes crashing down. Except the universe continues spinning and expanding regardless – our crashing consciousness is inconsequential either way.

This is, perhaps, one of the ways to understand what spiritual distress is. The amorality of our existence is laid bare, and everything is shaken. If nothing makes sense, then nothing makes sense. At these times, words often fail. (Language is contingent and constructed, too. When the bottom falls out of our presumption that we can depend on anything, for a time even the underpinnings of language are untethered and loose.)

Job was the only honest one in the story. In the end, everyone who tried to make sense of the tragedies or make Job feel better were Divinely declared wrong. The friends that said misfortune is the just result of sin and that God punishes the wicked were wrong. The friend who said Job's complaints and claims of innocence actually undermine religion was wrong. The friend who said Job should change his ways was wrong. Even God does not attempt to claim that creation makes sense. God's 129-verse long screed in reply to Job reads differently in light of this confession. The insanity is not in Job's umbrage at God. The insanity is the idea that the universe should correspond to human notions of justice and fairness at all.

This is bitter medicine to take. This is hard news. It does not square with how we see the world – normally. This ending was so uncomfortable, in fact, that later editors probably inserted the ending where Job's good fortune is doubled, and they also might have written in a backstory to justify Job's suffering as God 'testing' him. We just can't let senselessness be the end of the story! (Compare box office returns from Hollywood Rom-Coms versus any Ingmar Bergman film.)

But, maybe sometimes we should.

There is another element to this tale worth lifting up. Job is often pictured as the stoic, unshaken, resolved and faithful figure of supreme confidence in God's justice. Clearly, the bit about 'confidence in God's justice' is a deliberate (or even unconscious) re-cast of the story to make it more palatable to our human need to sense fairness. But the 'unshaken' reputation is also undeserved and unhelpful.

As early as chapter three (a mere 35 verses in), Job curses the day he was born. Later, he continues to complain: my suffering is undeserved and without end! "I loathe my life," he groans for 22 verses in chapter 10. "I am a laughingstock!" He cries out in anger, anguish, and despondent prayer: Make sense of this, God! "My spirit is broken," he says. "How long will you torment me?" Other people who don't deserve it are living well, while I am broken.

Reading through Job's responses to his friends reads like a script for most people in the midst of tragedy, trauma, and spiritual distress. The writer of this story put on Job's lips words of unimaginable pain. That they ring so true to our experience today demonstrates the deeply human phenomenon of spiritual distress. Job should be essential reading for anyone interested in working in this field – not because you believe in the Bible and not because you want a happy ending, but rather because it articulates the personal experience of spiritual distress from the inside, with an intimacy we rarely encounter in our happiness-addicted civilization. It also provides an understanding of how hollow conventional justifications sound – the platitudes or ham-handed attempts at soothing – when held up against the jarring reality of inexpressible tragedy.

Holding in mind the real gift of the book of Job is surprisingly hard. Our whole being revolts, so deeply is "fairness" written into our interpretation of the world. However, you will hear Job's words when sitting with people who are enduring profound loss, for whom the foundation of reality has been torn away.

There is, unfortunately, a common logical fallacy that clouds good judgment when struggling to find meaning in the midst of suffering. Humans seem hardwired to find meaning in things. That is a beautiful quality! Especially when that impulse seeks to transmute suffering into something valuable or informative that a person can take with them, this seems to be a natural healing mechanism our species depends on. We cannot help but try to find a 'silver lining,' make lemonade from lemons, find the good in the bad. We are creative enough to do it, too. We *do* create good out of bad.

Too often, though, then we then turn to 'the bad' and feel the need to say it wasn't bad after all. If we have this 'good' that we have fashioned, and that only could have resulted from the experience we had, then that experience must also have been 'good.' I find this line of reasoning dangerous and potentially abusive.

Allow me to illustrate this with an example I borrow from Dr. C. Robert Mesle, a professor of ethics and philosophy from my undergraduate alma mater. The human world was wracked for thousands of years by smallpox. This disease caused incalculable suffering and loss. It was, without a doubt, a 'bad' thing. It was, however, entirely eradicated from the planet with the development and deployment of a smallpox vaccine. Eliminating smallpox is definitely a 'good' thing. The whole world benefits from the invention and use of the smallpox vaccine. Since the smallpox vaccine is 'good,' and we wouldn't have the vaccine without smallpox, does that therefore mean that smallpox was actually 'good?'

You see the dilemma. How can we say a result of a thing is good, while the thing itself is bad? Does the goodness of the outgrowth change or outweigh the badness of the original problem it overcame?

We often describe how we acquired strengths or insights or perspectives through trials and struggles, that we otherwise couldn't imagine ourselves finding. It is so tempting, therefore, to view the struggles as themselves good or worthwhile. (Thinking of suffering as 'necessary' is a facet of this attempt at the redemption of suffering.) We might point to a child learning to walk (good) by falling down (bad). By this logic, however, a father who wants more good for his child should push his child down as often as he can while that little one is learning to walk. This is absurd, of course – no one would see that as kind or good.

I learned more from failing a particular exam in college than if I had passed it, true. But does that mean the F was 'good?' Should I have sought *more* Fs, so I could learn *more*? How much knowledge did I deny myself by struggling to get good grades?!

My wife and I learn more about our own individual psychologies and our shared relationship when we do not see eye to eye, even coming to a heated argument. Is marital strife actually good? Should I deliberately pick fights and try to argue more? Of course not.

Defeating Hitler and liberating the extermination camps was good. But no one will argue that Hitler was therefore actually a good man, and the extermination camps not profoundly evil.

Here is the rub. There is no logical necessity that our ability to create good from bad means that the bad was in fact good to begin with. We should allow ourselves and others the ability to call a bad thing 'bad,' even while acknowledging that we were able to create a good thing from the experience.

Humans are surprisingly good at making meaning out of suffering. This is a wonderful and valuable capacity. However, it does not follow that we should therefore call the suffering 'good.' Call a spade a spade. Allow evil to be known as evil. Allow suffering and injustice and absurdity to be just that. We can grow from it, surely. But our growth does not undo the injustice or necessitate us to endorse that thing.

Naturally, when working with individuals in distress, we should not be dissecting their comforting mechanisms or the logic of their belief systems. That would not be appropriate. In this work, we are not to impose our beliefs on others, even if we might personally disagree.

However, if someone seems to be struggling, perhaps feeling unconsciously beholden or forced to call the suffering 'good' in order to grow from it, recognizing the smallpox fallacy might be tremendously helpful for you and beneficial for the client. We do not have to say that what happened was good, in order to find good in our recovery from it. Like Job, we can let the bad be 'bad.' No need to back-peddle or obfuscate or soften or deny anything. Free the individual to embrace the goodness of their own growth, without having to deny the genuineness of their suffering.

Job's companions were not all bad. They were well-meaning, even if they were conventional and unimaginative. But they had one quality that redeems them forever in my estimation. When each of his three friends heard of Job's misfortunes, they set out to comfort and console him. When they finally found him – hardly recognizable, so distorted was he from his suffering – they tore their own robes as he had and sat in the dirt with him. They sat with him on the ground for *seven* days and nights before ever speaking a word of advice or consolation to him. For a full week, they simply listened to him and witnessed his grief. Only after this long time of nonjudgmental companioning were they able to appreciate how great his suffering was.

We can learn from their example. We do not need to run to justifications or excuses or palliatives that deny the genuineness of the pain, the unfairness, the non-sensical-ness, the horrific, hurtful insanity of it. Those denials are distractions at best and harmful at worst. One of the insights that might be gained is that experiences do not have to make sense to hurt, and the confrontation with a non-purposeful reality is part of the struggle and pain of spiritual distress. Denying it or acting as if that starkness is not real does not help people who are experiencing it. So, most of the tired, old lines just do not work. The prayer God answered, in the end, was Job's heartfelt, sincere denial of easy answers.

For all their faults, these were good friends who stuck with Job and listened far more than they spoke. I hope, when I am in sackcloth and ashes, I have similar companions who allow me to simply be in my grief for a good, long while. There is truth there.

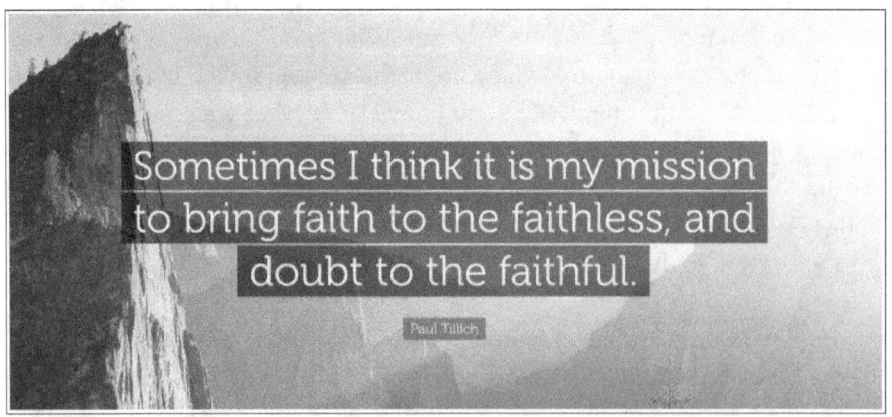

Sometimes I think it is my mission to bring faith to the faithless, and doubt to the faithful.

Paul Tillich

Appendix I:
Accessing the Spiritual Core of Hypnotism;
Hypnotism as Soul Medicine

Keynote for the Heartland Hypnosis Conference
April 29, 2023
The Rev. Dr. C. Scot Giles, DNGH

Hypnotism can be Soul Medicine. Clients often find the hypnotic process deeply meaningful, far more than simple counseling or psychotherapy. Many hypnotic practitioners report inexplicable flashes of insight when composing hypnotic material that turn out to be crucial to unlocking a client's problem. Much of this defies a purely rational explanation. Hypnotism works at the deepest level of the mind for both client and hypnotic operator, and can touch things that are profound and deeply spiritual. In this keynote address Dr. Giles explores how and why this happens, and how to cultivate it so that it happens more often.

———

Introduction

Good morning colleagues. For those of you who do not know me, I am not only a Consulting Hypnotist, but also a clergy person. I am a Unitarian Universalist minister in Full and Final Ministerial Fellowship, and a Board Certified Chaplain – a specialized training program for clergy who work in healthcare.

I am also a member of the Advisory Board of the National Guild of Hypnotists and the chairperson of its Ethics Committee. In the ranking structure of the Guild I am a Board Certified Diplomate. I have been in full-time hypnotic practice in the Chicagoland area for more than thirty-five years with a strong emphasis on hypnotic health coaching, mostly around issues related to cancer or fertility.

I have been interested in hypnotism from the time I was ten years old when I saw the great hypnotist Ormund McGill perform his Concert of Hypnotism on the Art Linkletter Show. I sent away for my first book on hypnotism which was advertised in the back of Superman Comics - using a graphic of a hypnotist in a tuxedo mesmerizing a voluptuous woman reclining on a couch wearing a dress she had put on using a brush and roller. There were lightening bolts coming out of the hypnotist's fingers. I would later learn that this graphic was actually done by Ormund McGill who owned a graphic design company at the time.

The book wasn't bad for something I saved up for by collecting quarters from my allowance to buy. The theory the book articulated we now know was false, but the basic techniques were the same as those taught in basic training today.

The book gave me everything I needed to get myself into trouble. I really did hypnotize my schoolmates to sing the Star Spangled Banner whenever the teacher turned her back to the class in order to erase the blackboard.

Yeah. That actually happened. I got in a ton of trouble and my parents forbade me from having anything to do with hypnotism going forward. You can see how well that worked.

I would grow up. I got formal training from some of the best. Became a hypnotist for real, but also a minister. My interest in spirituality is as deep as my interest in hypnotism. Therefore, I was pleased to receive the invitation to talk about the spiritual aspects of hypnotic practice here today.

The Spiritual Side

Reflecting on experiences I have had as a hypnotist, and those that colleagues have reported to me, when we do our hypnotic work with our clients, something else seems to happen. It is something that cannot be explained as resulting from hypnotic patter.

In this keynote I suggest that there are two things going on. First, the client may hear something the hypnotist did not say, and which spontaneously arises from the deeper mind of the client. That is a profound thing which guides the client towards individuation and wholeness. That certainly seems spiritual to me.

The second phenomenon is that the hypnotist, in deep rapport with the client, may spontaneously say just the right thing, often unplanned, that turns out to be the key to the client's unlocking. That is unquestionably a spiritual thing.

If you are in this profession long enough you will have the experience of something "more" manifesting in your hypnotic work that you may find hard to explain. This, I believe, shows that the hypnotic encounter actually has a spiritual aspect as well as a mental, physical and emotional aspect. There is a spiritual core to hypnotism. Hypnotism is Soul Medicine.

As hypnotic technicians, we know something about the way the human deeper mind works. For the purposes of this talk I will refer to that deeper part of the mind using the Ericksonian term, "unconsciousness." Others, who may embrace a different school of hypnotic thought may prefer to use the term "subconsciousness." That's fine. For the purposes of this address, I consider the unconscious and subconscious mind to be synonyms.

While there are some practitioners who simply ask a client what their goals are and confine the hypnotic work to a narrow focus on those specific goals, many practitioners (and I am one) will add a more general effort to help the client not just with specific goals, but also to achieve a higher level of functioning as a person.

Simply, while we work with the goals list in mind, we also want our clients to become better versions of themselves.

Some wag has said the secret to success in business is to under-promise and over-deliver. That is, to do more than is expected. I think that is true. Helping a client become a better version of themselves in an ethical way, as well as achieving the stated goals, is an example of being successful by doing more than is expected. Getting a reputation for doing that will give your practice long-term security because your clients get more than they came for in a good way.

The client may have come for weight control, smoking cessation, stress management or any of a number of other reasons. And I will address all of those concerns that the client may bring. But I also seek to get to know my clients as persons, and I always ask about how their life is going, and what they want for themselves in the longer term. And then I slip material intended to facilitate that into the work.

In my own practice, which has now spanned more than three decades, I have found this has paid huge benefits. And it is amplified by the two phenomena I mentioned and about which I have more to say.

Sneaky and Deceptive

I often remark that the reason there are so few hypnotists in practice isn't that there is a shortage of people who want to do it. No. Hypnotism instructors train a lot of people. Many instructors make most of their living teaching classes rather than working with individual clients. There should be a ton of hypnotists out there. But there are not.

I believe the reason there are so few hypnotists is that really good hypnotists are born, not made. That is, to really prosper in this profession you need to have a specific sort of personality. Those that have it do well, those that don't often move on to some other area of work or professional practice. We lack a calculus that can tell use which students will prosper and which will not, but in my experience that becomes obvious once a new hypnotist hangs out the shingle and gets to work.

I said this to a group of physicians when I was presenting to Grand Rounds at LaGrange Memorial Hospital some years ago (I had a program to help cancer patients with hypnotism based at that hospital for thirty years). One of the nurses raised her hand and asked, "So, Dr. Giles. What sort of personality does a hypnotist need to have?"

It may be a stain on my soul but I have a very dry sense of humor and so I replied "Well, you have to be a sneaky and deceptive person, willing to manipulate others with no compunction whatsoever." I got a round of laughter. But I was only half-kidding. There is something subversive about hypnotism, because you are subverting the client's resistance and any ill-formed defenses in order to help the client.

I mean the client already knows what they need to do. If you want to stop smoking, do not put a cigarette in your mouth and set it on fire. The client knows what to do. The problem is they can't bring themselves to do it. Our power is that we enlist their unconscious mind to impel them to do what they do not want to do, in order to achieve what they truly want to achieve.

Every successful hypnotist knows this. However, some of us go further. It's not just helping a client achieve a limited goal. We also help a client conduct a deeper appraisal of themselves and discover what they need to do to become more fulfilled as a person generally. In addition to helping with the specific goal, we also help them do a piece of interior work and become more fulfilled.

The Blueprint Hypothesis

Much of the work I do in my own hypnotic health coaching focuses on hypnotically enhanced fertility and on oncology (cancer care). At the core of the work I do are insights I learned from Dr. Bernie Siegel, with whom I have studied.

Born in 1932, Dr. Siegel was the Assistant Clinical Professor of General and Pediatric Surgery at Yale/New Haven Medical Center in Connecticut before he retired from medicine in 1989 to write books (he once told me his goal was to ultimately die of writer's cramp). He would come to found ECaP, or the Exceptional Cancer Patients Organization and I have taken their training program.

Dr. Siegel's first and best-known book is titled Love, Medicine and Miracles and was published in 1986. The book had a huge impact on me and was the reason I went to study with him. At its essence, Dr. Siegel's theory is that every human being has a spiritual core in their unconscious mind. That is, the deeper mind contains an image of who that person should be.

Depending on your theology you might think this image, which I will call the "inner blueprint," might be a gift from a spiritual power. But some of the colleagues who trained with me thought that previous lives and reincarnation may play a role. Others believed it is something that arises from a Collective Unconsciousness that we all share together. What one believes doesn't matter.

The empirical finding is that everyone appears to have an inner blueprint for who they were created to be. To the degree that a person figures out their inner blueprint and creates a life for themselves that captures some of that inner plan, is the degree to which that person will be happy and fulfilled. And, as Dr. Siegel found, that is the degree to which they become physically and emotionally resilient to life-changing medical problems like cancer or other aliments.

To the degree that a person has not actualized their inner blueprint in their day-to-day lives is the degree to which their physical and emotional resilience is flawed. They appear to become susceptible to a whole range of medical and emotional problems. Dr. Siegel found that if you can help a person discover what their inner blueprint is, then they would not only do better medically, but also in every other arena of their life. That is a holistic focus. That is Soul Medicine.

Dr. Siegel developed a program using a support groups, guided imagery and self-hypnotism as well as dream and drawing interpretation to help people look for and understand their inner blueprint.

People often have no idea of what the inner blueprint in their unconscious mind for themselves might be. Usually they start out their lives with some clues – childhood fantasies, heroes in movies or literature, their own remembered dreams. But far too often people move away from that inner guidance because it seems impractical.

So the person who was supposed to be a poet becomes an accountant, because that is easier. The person who really wanted to be a chef becomes an insurance salesperson instead, because they discovered that culinary work doesn't pay well. But the inner urge is still there, and if no way can be found to move toward it, at least to some degree, frustration builds and resilience plummets.

For thirty years at LaGrange Memorial Hospital in LaGrange, Illinois I ran a program called I Can Act Now (abbreviated ICAN). It was the first medically approved, hospital based program in the United States for hypnotic interventions into cancer.

Because we were based at a single institution for three decades we were able to follow our participants. If you are curious you will find an analysis of our findings in the download directory of my website. (Also available here: https://ngh.net/ten-year-study-of-using-hypnosis-for-people-living-with-cancer/) But briefly, we showed that adding hypnotism to conventional medical care produced, reliably and over time, improved outcomes when our participants' results were compared to the national cancer outcomes database.

Yet, other programs of doing hypnotism with people who were living with cancer, such as the original programs by Dr. O. Carl Simonton, did not produce this sort of result. I suspect the reason is that the other programs confined their focus to specific problems – nausea, loss of appetite, discomfort, etc. We covered those bases too, but we also included the search for the inner blueprint in all of the hypnotic work we did. That is what, I believe, did the trick. We didn't just work with symptoms. We looked for the spiritual core and helped our participants find it.

I'm encouraged in this belief by noticing that many of the other approaches, including the more recent work of those following Dr. Simonton, have been evolving in exactly this direction – perhaps proving that all worthwhile helping techniques tend to converge over time.

So how does one help a client find their inner blueprint? I suggest there are two tools we use which plumb the deepest level of the client's mind, and also that of the hypnotist. These are spiritual tools.

Spirituality and the Unconscious Mind

I believe that spirituality, the sense of connection between oneself and something greater, arises in the unconscious process.

This is an insight that comes from depth psychology. The great analyst Dr. Carl Jung based his whole therapeutic system on helping his patients discover who they were supposed to be, as opposed to who events had made them become. He identified that process as the core of his therapy. Further, he believed that the unconscious mind of one person was connected at a deep level to a Collective Unconsciousness which contains a wisdom and a structure that we all have access to.

I have come to agree. My evidence for this comes from a phenomena I have observed as a minister and as a hypnotist. I call it "Hearing A Word No Mouth Has Spoken."

As a minister I have delivered many sermons. It is not uncommon to have someone come up after and say something like, "That was fantastic. It changed my life! You have to give me a copy of what you said."

So you give them a copy. Then, later you ask if they received it. And they say, "Yeah, but it wasn't the right one." But it was the right one. They heard something in the sermon that was not actually there. They were ready to have an insight or awareness, and their unconscious mind used the occasion of my sermon to let that awareness manifest in their mind. They thought it was something I said. But it was not. It was something they said, to themselves. I just provided the occasion for their unconscious mind to guide them.

This phenomena has been known for a very long time. In the spiritual classic, the Tao Te Ching the ancient sage Lao Tzu wrote "when the student is ready the teacher will appear."

He didn't mean that there was a celestial backlog of insightful teachers, and somehow one would be supplied to a seeker on a schedule by an Amazon delivery driver.

He meant that when the mind is ready to have an insight, it will find a way to let that insight manifest. My parishioner was ready to understand something about themselves. In the words of my sermon the parishioner found a way to manifest that insight. They did the work. My sermon just provided the opportunity, because I did not actually say what they heard. They heard a word no mouth had spoken.

Well, hypnotic work with a client can do exactly the same thing. Many of us will have the experience of a client reporting how wonderfully our hypnotic work helped them, how insightful they found our words, and how as a result of the session whole new areas of their lives were pulling together or taking a new direction.

When this first happened to me I said to myself, "Wow! I must be really good at this." The trouble was when I listened to the recording I'd made of the session I realized that I had never said anything intended to cause changes like that in my client's life. But the session did cause that change. Not because of anything I did, but because the client had heard something I did not need to say. What the client heard came from the client's deeper mind, or their soul, if you prefer. It did not come from me.

The student was ready. The teacher appeared. The teacher wasn't the hypnotist. the teacher was the unconscious mind of the client who heard in the hypnotist's words something the client needed to hear. The hypnotist was just the vehicle.

The hypnotist allows the client to discover something the client knows at the unconscious level, and that allows the possibility that the client will make it real.

This is a profound thing, and many would call that level of profundity a spiritual thing. I do. Yet essentially I am describing a psychological phenomena – the client gives birth to an awareness from their own unconscious mind. Certainly it has a spiritual aspect in that it can be deeply moving, but the action is occurring within the psychology of the client him or herself.

Spirituality implies something more than a purely psychological phenomenon. While the client realizing something profound about themselves may in fact arise from a power deeper than their own mind, there is something more.

Transpersonal Spirituality

There is more going on at a spiritual level in the hypnotic consultation than just what I have said so far and builds upon it.

Every hypnotist knows that what makes hypnotism effective is not just the hypnotic induction itself. What adds the power is that the hypnotic induction occurs in the context of a relationship between hypnotist and client. If the hypnotist does their work well, they will have excellent rapport building skills and forge a powerful connection with the client. This is what Ericksonian hypnotist Dr. Stephen Gilligan calls "the Cooperation Principle." The hypnotist and client enter into a mutually transformative relationship, cooperating together on the common goal of helping the client.

Yes, I did say the relationship is "mutually transformative." You will find that as a person you change when you start to practice as a hypnotist. In order to achieve the sort of deep rapport good hypnotic work requires you will find yourself changing. In order to work with someone who is quite different from yourself you will need to call into question and rethink things you had believed or not understood fully. The hypnotist helps the client change. The client helps the hypnotist change.

In 1991 Grove Press published a book titled Doctor Sleep by Madison Smartt Bell. If you don't know the book I do recommend it, as the story is told from the perspective of a working hypnotist who moved to London to set up a practice and escape a troubled past. At one point he is hypnotizing his client and he actually nods off into self-hypnotic trance himself in the middle of his hypnotic patter.

That is something that has happened to more than a few of us, I know.

In the story the hypnotist was startled to hear himself insert into his patter something he had not planned to say, but it turned out to be exactly what his client needed to hear to trigger a healing insight.

In this case it wasn't exactly the client "hearing a word no mouth had spoken," because the hypnotist did speak it. But there was no reason for him to have done so. The words came drifting up out of his unconscious mind because of a connection that existed between himself and his client.

Brought to the fore by the hypnotic rapport, the unconscious minds of the hypnotist and client were, I propose, linked through a collective awareness and a shared wisdom came to be. The words the hypnotist said in the patter actually didn't amount to much, but somehow in a shared state of consciousness, something emerged that cannot be explained as mere psychological connection.

Hypnotism and Spiritual Consciousness

Most hypnotic inductions involve some sort of synchronization to the client's breathing rhythm. Different systems do it differently but often one will count the client down in time to the client's breath, or one will parse suggestions so they are recited in time to the client's respiration. This is a standard technique, used since the time of Mesmer.

Yet, the next time you do it pay attention to your own breathing as you work with your client. I find, as have most of those I have taught, that you will regulate your own breathing in time with the client. During the hypnotic induction, very often the subject and operator are in sync. They breathe in unison, words flow in time to the beat of the breath.

As a clergy person and chaplain, as someone trained in spiritual techniques from around the world, I can point you to systems of spiritual development all over the globe where exactly this technique is used.

The shaman chants in rhythm to the supplicant's breath. The Russian Orthodox *Starets* (one of whom, by the way, was Rasputin) recites prayers in rhythm to his or her breathing in the monastery or convent, and when in a group, the whole group breathes as one. The Dessert Mothers and Fathers of Christianity taught the importance (in 1Thessalonians 5:17) of "pray without ceasing," which meant to pray while breathing. The Buddhist and Sufi Meditation Masters teach much the same thing, as does the yoga adept.

It is said that on average, you will take a billion breaths in your lifetime. Your breathing does more than just oxygenate your blood. While your heartbeat is controlled by a pacemaker (natural or artificial) located within the organ of the heart itself, your breathing is controlled by your brain.

The ancient Greek physician Galen noted that gladiators whose necks were broken at the angle to damage their brain stem could no longer breathe. We now call the part of the brain stem that controls this the pre-Bötzinger Complex. The brain-breath connection works in both directions. If you damage the brain, breathing can be stopped. But if you control the breathing, you also change the brain. Every advance-level martial artist learns breathing rhythms that overcome fatigue, quiet fear, improve clarity of mind and boost an awareness of what the opponent might do next.

Modern science teaches us the value of mindfulness meditation, a sort of present-moment focus that is created by centering attention on the breath.

While the technique has been known for centuries, the medical value of the practice has been documented in our time. Dr. Jon Kabat-Zinn wrote about the technique in his book Full Catastrophe Living after teaching it at the University of Massachusetts Medical Center, and Mindfullness Based Stress Management is now taught in hospitals around the nation.

I believe all of these spiritual techniques amount to Hypnotism Lite. What we do with our clients in our consultation rooms is a more powerful and structured version of what spiritual directors and teachers the world over have been doing since time immemorial.

Those same spiritual directors and teachers talk about how, in the deep inner place that breath work brings them to, they sense a connection to something larger than themselves. Some call this something "God." Some call it "Buddha Consciousness." Hermetic practitioners call it "Cosmic Consciousness." The Sufi call it "Nearness to Allah." Psychologist William James called it "Something More." Dr. Carl Jung called it the "Collective Unconsciousness."

Call it what you will. That many people describing what is obviously the same thing, are unlikely to be wrong. There is a deeper something that is contacted during the immense rapport of the inner state of mind that hypnotism can harness and during which "Something More" becomes manifest. And the hypnotist finds themselves saying exactly what needs to be said to meet the hunger in the client for meaning. And the hypnotist often does not know why.

Ah...but the result is there. The key to the client's opening is found. The client discovers what their deepest desires are, and resolves to somehow manifest a part of the inner blueprint.

Like "Hearing A Word No Mouth Has Spoken," this is a profound thing. But it is also a thing that transcends the individual psychology of the client. Something more has manifested in the deep rapport of subject and hypnotic operator.

If that is not a spiritual connection, I do not know what is.

The Complete Hypnotist

Sadly, not every hypnotic practitioner gets good at this. But many do. The best do.

As a hypnotist of many decades standing I believe one can sort of tell, and one can get a sense of what the hallmarks are of those who are good at this. Here is what I have noticed.

The best hypnotists, the colleagues who practice Soul Medicine, work with clients.

That may seem odd, but you'd be surprised how many colleagues out there have abandoned client work and while teaching classes about hypnotism, have ceased to practice it themselves. Perhaps they have gone as deep as they can go in their own self-transformation. Perhaps they no longer care. Perhaps money has become more important to them than helping. But you can tell. After a time what they have to teach feels shop-worn and dusty. They have lost passion. The best hypnotists work with clients, at least some of the time.

The best hypnotists, the Soul Doctors (if you will) regularly practice self-hypnotism in one of its many forms.

Simply, they do their own inner work. They attempt to deal with there own stuff – their traumas, resentments, hurts and pain. They learn by regular practice how to self-sooth and as a result become deeper and wiser people themselves. In hypnotism, more than in any other helping profession, what you do has to be who you are. Your methodology needs to flow from your personality and temperament. If you don't have yourself together, your clients can tell and they will not trust you to accompany them to the deeper realms. You can't take your client to a place you have never been.

In Conclusion

We are all works in progress. I look back with chagrin at some of my early hypnotic work and realize that I'm so much better now. That's okay. I hope I keep learning and becoming better as a hypnotist until the moment I leave this world. We never know it all and there is always something new to learn.

But I want to make my hypnotic practice Soul Medicine. I want to stay in touch with the spiritual core of the hypnotic arts and sciences. I hope you agree. For there are rewards – to both you and your clients – for so doing.

And that is what I have to share with you in this keynote today. I hope you have a fantastic conference experience.

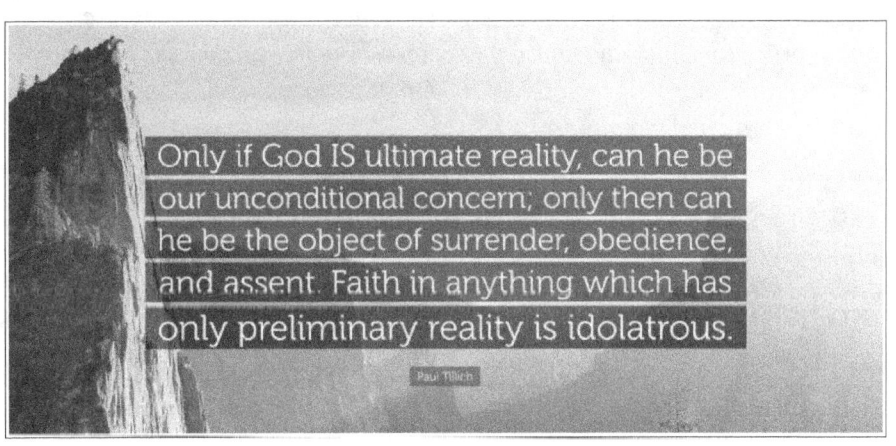

Only if God IS ultimate reality, can he be our unconditional concern; only then can he be the object of surrender, obedience, and assent. Faith in anything which has only preliminary reality is idolatrous.

Paul Tillich

Appendix II:
Psychotherapists or the Clergy – Carl Jung

What follows is an excerpt from a speech that Carl G. Jung, the Swiss psychologist and pioneer of Analytical Psychology, gave to a gathering of Swiss clergy in 1932. While there are specific Christian references and the language is dated, this selection nevertheless speaks of universal themes and enduring insight about the importance of tending to clients' souls (the original meaning of 'psyche') as well as their physiology. Not one to simply endorse 'business as usual,' however, Jung also challenged his audience to recognize that in order to genuinely minister to people, they must acknowledge, accept, and love those parts of themselves they might want to condemn or hide for fear of others' condemnation.

The speech as a whole merits consideration, and is available in its entirety on the NGH Clergy Special Interest Group website (www.ngh-csig.net). However, most significant for our purposes are paragraphs 519-526, reproduced below in slightly adapted/updated form.

From *Psychology and Religion West and East,* Collected Works of Carl G. Jung, Vol. II

People forget that even clinicians have moral scruples and that certain client's confessions are hard even for a clinician to swallow yet the patient does not feel themselves accepted unless the very worst in them is accepted too. No one can bring this about by mere words. It comes only through reflection and through the clinician's attitude towards themselves and their own dark side.

If the clinician wants to guide another, or even accompany them a step of the way, they must feel with that person's psyche. One never feels it when one passes judgment. Whether one puts one's judg-

ments into words or keeps them to oneself makes not the slightest difference. To take the opposite position and to agree with the client offhand is also of no use. Feeling comes only through unprejudiced objectivity.

This sounds almost like a scientific precept and it could be confused with a purely intellectual, abstract attitude of mind, but what I mean is something quite different. It is a human quality, a kind of deep respect for the facts, for the one who suffers from them, and for the riddle of such a person's life.

The truly religious person has this attitude; one knows that God has brought all sorts of strange and inconceivable things to pass and seeks in the most curious ways to enter a person's heart. One therefore senses in everything the unseen presence of the divine will. This is what I mean by unprejudiced objectivity. It is a moral achievement on the part of the clinician who ought not to let themselves be repelled by sickness and corruption.

We cannot change anything unless we accept it. Condemnation does not liberate, it oppresses. I am the oppressor of the person I condemn, not his friend and fellow sufferer. I do not in the least mean to say that we must never pass judgment when we desire to help and improve. But, if the clinician wishes to help a human being, they must be able to accept the client as they are and one can do this, in reality, only when one has already seen and accepted themselves as they are.

Perhaps this sounds very simple but simple things are always the most difficult. In actual life, it requires the greatest art to be simple. And so, acceptance of oneself is the essence of the moral problem and the acid test of one's whole outlook on life. That I feed the beggar, that I forgive an insult, that I love my enemy in the name of Christ – all these are undoubtedly great virtues. What I do unto the least of my brethren, that I do unto Christ. But what if I should discover that the least amongst them all, the poorest of all beggars, the most impudent of all offenders, yay the very fiend himself, that these are within me, and that I myself stand in need of my own kindness, that I myself am the enemy whom must be loved, what then?

Then, as a rule, the whole truth of Christianity is reversed. There is then no more talk of love and long suffering. We say to the despicable brother within us, "Raka!", and condemn and rage against ourselves. We hide that part from the world. We deny ever having met this least among the lowly in ourselves and had it been God himself who drew near to us in this despicable form we should have denied that part a thousand times before a single cock had crowed.

Healing may be called a religious problem. In the sphere of social or national relations, the state of suffering may be civil war and this state is to be cured by the Christian virtue of forgiveness and love of one's enemies. That which we recommend with the conviction of good Christians as applicable to external situations we must also apply inwardly in the treatment of neurosis. This is why modern humanity has heard enough about guilt and sin. They are sorely beset by their own bad conscience and want rather to know how they are to reconcile themselves with their own nature, how they are to love the enemy in their own heart and call the wolf their own kind.

Modern humanity does not want to know in what way they can imitate Christ but in what way they can live their own individual lives, however meager and uninteresting they may be. It is because every form of imitation seems to them deadening and sterile that they rebel against the force of tradition that would hold them to well-trodden ways. All such roads, for modern sensibilities, lead in the wrong direction.

One may not know it, but one behaves as if one's own individual life were God's special Will which must be fulfilled at all costs. This is the source of one's egoism, which is one of the most tangible evils of the neurotic state. But the person who tells someone they are too egoistic has already lost their confidence, and rightly so, for that person has driven them still further into their neurosis.

If I wish to affect a cure for my clients, I am forced to acknowledge the deep significance of their egoism. I should be blind indeed if I did not recognize it as a true will of God. I must even help the client to prevail in their egoism. If they succeed in this, they estrange themselves from other people, they drive others away and the others come to themselves, as they should, for they were seeking to rob the client of their sacred egoism! This must be left to client, for it is their strongest and healthiest power.

It is a true will of God that sometimes drives them into complete isolation. However wretched this state may be, it also stands one in good stead, for in this way alone can one get to know oneself and learn what an invaluable treasure is the love of one's fellow beings. It is, moreover, only in the state of complete abandonment and loneliness that we experience the helpful powers of our own natures.

Appendix III:
Competencies for Addressing Spiritual and Religious Issues in Counseling
by the American Counseling Association

*Consulting Hypnotists are not Counselors, of course, and unless li-
censed for such work we should always be cognizant of the limits of our scope
of practice. Including the following document in this book should not be con-
strued as an endorsement of Spiritual Hypnotism Providers, in themselves, as
anything more than specially trained consulting hypnotists. Some of the
points enumerated below (such as diagnosis or treatment) use language that
is out of scope for most hypnotists and may be irrelevant for unlicensed practitioner. However, that having been said, the American Counseling Association
has prepared this list of competencies for counselors doing work in this area.
Even if they are not directly applicable, these competencies identify expectations for professionals working in this field. This is helpful perspective as a
general orientation to competencies professional Spiritual Hypnotism
Providers should aspire to.*

*As always, hypnotists should hold themselves to the highest interpre-
tation of the NGH Code of Ethics and all legal responsibilities in their respec-
tive state or nation. Beyond that, hypnotists interested in offering hypnosis for
spiritual distress might consult the following for direction regarding further
training, orientation, or personal and professional development. It is in this
spirit that the following is reproduced in this volume.*

Preamble

The Competencies for Addressing Spiritual and Religious Issues in
Counseling are guidelines that complement, not supersede, the values and
standards espoused in the ACA Code of Ethics. Consistent with the ACA
Code of Ethics (2005), the purpose of the ASERVIC Competencies is to "rec-

ognize diversity and embrace a cross-cultural approach in support of the worth, dignity, potential, and uniqueness of people within their social and cultural contexts" (p. 3). These Competencies are intended to be used in conjunction with counseling approaches that are evidence-based and that align with best practices in counseling. This Preamble must accompany any publication or dissemination, in whole or in part, of the ASERVIC Competencies.

Culture and Worldview

1. The professional counselor can describe the similarities and differences between spirituality and religion, including the basic beliefs of various spiritual systems, major world religions, agnosticism, and atheism.

2. The professional counselor recognizes that the client's beliefs (or absence of beliefs) about spirituality and/or religion are central to his or her worldview and can influence psychosocial functioning.

Counselor Self-Awareness

3. The professional counselor actively explores his or her own attitudes, beliefs, and values about spirituality and/or religion.

4. The professional counselor continuously evaluates the influence of his or her own spiritual and/or religious beliefs and values on the client and the counseling process.

5. The professional counselor can identify the limits of his or her understanding of the client's spiritual and/or religious perspective and is acquainted with religious and spiritual resources and leaders who can be avenues for consultation and to whom the counselor can refer.

Human and Spiritual Development

6. The professional counselor can describe and apply various models of spiritual and/or religious development and their relationship to human development.

Communication

7. The professional counselor responds to client communications about spirituality and/or religion with acceptance and sensitivity.

8. The professional counselor uses spiritual and/or religious concepts that are consistent with the client's spiritual and/or religious perspectives and are acceptable to the client.

9. The professional counselor can recognize spiritual and/or religious themes in client communication and is able to address these with the client when they are therapeutically relevant.

Assessment

10. During the intake and assessment processes, the professional counselor strives to understand a client's spiritual and/or religious perspective by gathering information from the client and/or other sources.

Diagnosis and Treatment

11. When making a diagnosis, the professional counselor recognizes that the client's spiritual and/or religious perspectives can a) enhance well-being; b) contribute to client problems; and/or c) exacerbate symptoms.

12. The professional counselor sets goals with the client that are consistent with the client's spiritual and/or religious perspectives.

13. The professional counselor is able to a) modify therapeutic techniques to include a client's spiritual and/or religious perspectives, and b) utilize spiritual and/or religious practices as techniques when appropriate and acceptable to a client's viewpoint.

14. The professional counselor can therapeutically apply theory and current research supporting the inclusion of a client's spiritual and/or religious perspectives and practices.

Revised and Approved, 5/5/2009 ©ASERVIC 5/5/09 NOTE: The American Counseling Association (ACA) has now endorsed The Spiritual Competencies

Appendix IV:
Defining Spiritual Distress

Excerpted from
"An Integrative Review of Defining Characteristics of the Nursing Diagnosis 'Spiritual Distress'"
By Fateme Eshghi, Lida Nikfarid, Armin Zareiyan

Nursing Open, *10*(5),2023, pp. 2831-2841

Introduction

In recent decades, health-related disciplines have paid remarkable attention to the issue of spirituality, as evidenced by the growing trend of publishing research and theoretical articles on the subject of spirituality and related concepts (Bornet et al., 2016). In line with the reported positive impact of spirituality on health, other reports have focused on the relationship between spirituality and the negative consequences of illness and hardships of life (de Oliveira Maraldi, 2020; Monod et al., 2010; Smucker, 1996; Tanyi, 2002). According to evidence, some people have feelings such as being punished, being purified, and guilty in the experiences like disasters and crises (Sipon et al., 2015; Tanyi, 2002). According to researches neglecting the patient's spiritual needs can lead to feelings of isolation and spiritual distress (Narayanasamy, 2006). North American Nursing Diagnosis Association-International (NANDA-I) introduced spiritual distress as a nursing diagnosis in 1978. Then, in the last version (2018–2020), spiritual distress was defined as a state of suffering related to impaired ability to experience meaning-giving in life, through connection to self, others, the world and nature, and a superior being (Ackley et al., 2021). The NANDA-I describes responses of persons to identified health problems as *the defining characteristics* of nursing diagnoses (Assis et al., 2018; Carpenito-Moyet, 2006).

Background

Religious and spiritual values and attitudes of people are challenged in times of illness and loss. These beliefs include their meaning given to life, sense of hope, and faith. Consequently, the person may experience a sense of doubt, confusion, and tension (Kord & Biadar, 2019; Koslander et al., 2021; Mrdjenovich, 2019). Concepts such as religious struggle, spiritual stress, and religious anguish thus found their way into health care providers' literature. Spiritual distress happens when persons are at risk of experiencing disruption in their value and belief system, which are the cause of hope, strength, and the meaning of life for them. In this case, the persons may need specialized care considerations provided by healthcare providers to prevent negative consequences such as reduced quality of life, less personal satisfaction, and wellness (Hatamipour et al., 2018; Narayanasamy, 2006).

The dependence of culture and religion on spirituality is one of the main reasons for the numerous studies done to validate the diagnosis of spiritual distress nursing (Erickson & Carlson, 2014). Research has recently looked at the prevalence of spiritual distress and emphasized prioritizing it.

Considering that spiritual distress is a complex, abstract and multi-dimensional phenomenon influenced by the cultural and religious context of the individual, determining the criteria that accurately define spiritual distress is an important issue. Nursing care should be in line with culture and religion. This integrated review was designed to determine the defining characteristics of spiritual distress as the first step of a validation study, as the integrated review demonstrates a more comprehensive understanding and knowledge of the phenomenon.

This review extracted the most frequent defining characteristics in the resources. Lack of peace, a sense of hopelessness, changes in anger behaviour, changes in the meaning given to life, fear, frequent crying, and disturbance in the system of beliefs were of them.

The **lack of peace** (Caldeira et al., 2013; Caldeira et al., 2014; Caldeira et al., 2016; Caldeira et al., 2017b; Chaves, Carvalho, & Hass, 2010; Chaves, Carvalho, Terra, & Souza, 2010; Hatamipour et al., 2015; Ku et al., 2010; Schultz et al., 2018; Simão et al., 2015) and **lack of hope** (Caldeira et al., 2013; Caldeira et al., 2017a; Chaves, Carvalho, & Hass, 2010; Chaves, Carvalho, Terra, & Souza, 2010; Glenn & Pieper, 2019; Hatamipour et al., 2015; Martins & Caldeira, 2018; Pinho et al., 2017; Simão et al., 2015; Yang et al., 2012) were the most common defining characteristics mentioned in almost half of the reviewed studies. Both of these characteristics were related to the subcategory of spiritual suffering concerning the self. In the study of Caldeira et al, it was concluded that lack of peace and hope were the most common defining characteristics of spiritual distress(Caldeira et al., 2013). Hatamipour et al., in their qualitative study, aimed at determining the spiritual needs of cancer patients, named **peace-seeking** as one of the main themes. In this study, hope was the subcategory of the peace-seeking theme (Hatamipour et al., 2015). Lopez Chaves et al., in their study, stated that lack of peace (Chaves, Carvalho, & Hass, 2010; Chaves, Carvalho, Terra, & Souza, 2010) and **lack of hope** (Chaves, Carvalho, Terra, & Souza, 2010) are the most important defining characteristics with a high frequency. According to Caldeira, lack of peace is a major defining characteristic of nursing diagnosis spiritual distress (Caldeira et al., 2016). Schultz et al. reported the **lack of inner peace** as one of the main statements of spiritual distress (Schultz et al., 2018).

In their study, Velosa et al. (2017) reported that patients with spiritual distress as a nursing diagnosis have more than one defining characteristic; and **anger behavior** was one of the most important characteristics. In a clinical validation study on impaired spirituality, anger behavior was the most common characteristic (Chaves, Carvalho, Terra, & Souza, 2010).

Pinho et al., reported a **lack of meaning in life** and **asking the meaning of life**, along with the **lack of purpose**, as the major defining characteristics of spiritual distress (Pinho et al., 2017). In Chaves's study, the lack of meaning in life ranked third among the other seven most important defining characteristics of spiritual distress (Chaves, Carvalho, & Hass, 2010). They reported the lack of meaning in life as one of the defining characteristics of spiritual distress in patients with chronic diseases (Chaves, Carvalho, Terra, & Souza, 2010). Hatamipour et al., in their qualitative study based on interviews with cancer patients, extracted this characteristic as one of the main themes (Hatamipour et al., 2015). Caldeira et al., reported asking the meaning of life as one of the major defining characteristics of spiritual distress (Caldeira et al., 2016; Caldeira et al., 2017a). But in the other study, the lack of meaning of life was reported as a minor defining characteristic of spiritual distress (Caldeira et al., 2017a).

In the studies conducted by Caldeira et al., **behavior change, fear, and crying**, along with ten other characteristics, were reported as major criteria for spiritual distress (Caldeira et al., 2016; Caldeira et al., 2017a). Also, they mentioned these two criteria as defining characteristics of spiritual distress in their integrated review, these two criteria were mentioned along with other criteria as defining characteristics of spiritual distress (Caldeira et al., 2013).

Concern about the belief system or God has been reported in several studies as a defining characteristic of spiritual distress (Caldeira et al., 2013; Glenn & Pieper, 2019; Monod et al., 2010; Monod et al., 2012; Simão et al., 2015). In the qualitative research of Hatamipour et al., strengthening spiritual beliefs, communication with God, and prayer, as subcategories of the **theme of transcendence**, were from the spiritual needs of cancer patients (Hatamipour et al., 2015). In the study of Chaves et al., concern about the belief system and/or God was reported as the first and most important criterion among the seven main defining characteristics of the nursing diagnosis of spiritual distress. They reported this characteristic with a frequency of 27.3% has little correlation with the nursing diagno-sis of spiritual distress. However, the researchers in this study stated that they extracted this criterion, along with several other characteristics, through an integrated review of literature, as the first step of their research (Chaves, Carvalho, Terra, & Souza, 2010). Caldeira et al., reported similar re-sults and concluded that this characteristic was irrelevant to the nursing di-agnosis of spiritual distress (Caldeira et al., 2017a). This criterion was com-mon in our integrated review study. On the other hand, other studies have reported conflicting results about this criterion as defining characteristic of the nursing diagnosis of spiritual distress. Therefore, it is necessary to con-duct other quantitative and qualitative studies taking into account the views of patients and experts in the field of spirituality to identify the phenome-non of spiritual distress as much as possible and provide specific high-qual-ity care for it. It should be noted that this contradiction can be due to differ-ent samples or cultural and religious backgrounds of the people participat-ing in the studies.

Conclusion

According to the findings of this study, lack of peace, hopelessness, anger, change in the meaning given to life, fear, and crying were the most defining features in the reviewed texts for the diagnosis of spiritual distress nursing. *(**Note from Editor**: "concern about God" was mentioned above as a key quality of spiritual distress in several studies, but as often as 1/3 of the time was not experienced by patients otherwise qualifying for the diagnosis. So, "concern about belief system or God" was not included by these authors in the defining features for spiritual distress. It might be appropriate for you, as a hypnotist-clinician, to consider for yourself the place of "concern about God" in your conception of spiritual distress, as well as recognizing that there is scholarly disagreement about its validity for a nursing diagnosis. The key takeaway for hypnotists working with spiritual distress is that one cannot as-sume "concern about God" is being experienced by someone experiencing spir-itual distress, and more follow-up is required.)*

As a result, these defining characteristics can lead clinicians to con-sider the nursing diagnosis of spiritual distress for their patients. Determi-nation of the defining characteristics that most likely present a nursing di-agnosis facilitates the provision of appropriate and individualized care. The emphasized view of holistic care in nursing necessitates attention to the spiritual dimension of care as much attention to spiritual care as it does to other aspects of human health.

The excerpt above has been used under Creative Commons license, edited (sections selected) and adapted (some spelling and grammar correc-tions) for relevance to hypnotists.

References

Ackley, B. J., Ladwig, G. B., Makic, M. B. F., Martinez-Kratz, M., & Zanotti, M. (2021). *Nursing diagnosis handbook, revised reprint with 2021–2023 NANDA-I® updates-E-Book*. Elsevier Health Sciences.

Assis, G. L. C. d., Sousa, C. S., Turrini, R. N. T., Poveda, V. d. B., & Silva, R. d. C. G. (2018). Proposal of nursing diagnoses, outcomes and interventions for postoperative patients of orthognathic surgery. *Revista da Escola de Enfermagem da USP*, 52, e03321.

Bornet, M.-A., Rochat, E., Dürst, A.-V., Fustinoni, S., Büla, C., von Gunten, A., & Monod, S. (2016). Instruments to assess depressive symptoms and spiritual distress investigate different dimensions. *Clinical Gerontologist*, 39, 104–116.

Caldeira, S., Carvalho, E. C., & Vieira, M. (2013). Spiritual distress—Proposing a new definition and defining characteristics. *International Journal of Nursing Knowledge*, 24, 77–84.

Caldeira, S., Carvalho, E. C. d., & Vieira, M. (2014). Between spiritual wellbeing and spiritual distress: Possible related factors in elderly patients with cancer. *Revista Latino-Americana de Enfermagem*, 22, 28–34.

Caldeira, S., Timmins, F., de Carvalho, E. C., & Vieira, M. (2016). Nursing diagnosis of "spiritual distress" in women with breast cancer: Prevalence and major defining characteristics. *Cancer Nursing*, 39, 321–327.

Caldeira, S., Timmins, F., de Carvalho, E. C., & Vieira, M. (2017a). Clinical validation of the nursing diagnosis spiritual distress in cancer patients undergoing chemotherapy. *International Journal of Nursing Knowledge*, 28, 44–52.

Caldeira, S., Timmins, F., de Carvalho, E. C., & Vieira, M. (2017b). Spiritual well-being and spiritual distress in cancer patients undergoing chemotherapy: Utilizing the SWBQ as component of holistic nursing diagnosis. *Journal of Religion and Health*, 56, 1489–1502.

Carpenito-Moyet, L. J. (2006). *Nursing diagnosis: Application to clinical practice*. Lippincott Williams & Wilkins.

Chaves, E. d. C. L., Carvalho, E., & Hass, V. J. J. A. P. d. E. V. (2010). Validation of the nursing diagnosis spiritual anguish: Analysis by experts. *Acta Paulista de Enfermagem*, 23, 264–270.

Chaves, E. d. C. L., Carvalho, E. C. d., Terra, F. d. S., & Souza, L. d. (2010). Clinical validation of impaired spirituality in patients with chronic renal disease. *Revista Latino-Americana de Enfermagem*, 18, 309–316.

de Oliveira Maraldi, E. (2020). Response bias in research on religion, spirituality and mental health: A critical review of the literature and methodological recommendations. *Journal of Religion and Health*, 59, 772–783.

Erickson, M. J., & Carlson, T. (2014). *Spirituality and family therapy*. Routledge.

Glenn, C. T., & Pieper, B. (2019). Forgiveness and spiritual distress: Implications for nursing. *Journal of Christian Nursing*, 36, 185–189.

Hatamipour, K., Rassouli, M., Yaghmaie, F., Zendedel, K., & Alavi Majd, H. (2018). Development and psychometrics of a 'spiritual needs assessment scale of patients with cancer': A mixed exploratory study. *International Journal of Cancer Management*, 11, e10083.

Hatamipour, K., Rassouli, M., Yaghmaie, F., Zendedel, K., & Majd, H. A. (2015). Spiritual needs of cancer patients: A qualitative study. *Indian Journal of Palliative Care*, 21, 61–67.

Kord, B., & Biadar, S. (2019). Predictive role of spiritual well-being for optimism and life expectancy among women who referred to health centers. *Health, Spirituality and Medical Ethics*, 6, 23–28.

Koslander, T., Rönning, S., Magnusson, S., & Wiklund Gustin, L. (2021). A 'near-life experience': Lived experiences of spirituality from the perspective of people who have been subject to inpatient psychiatric care. *Scandinavian Journal of Caring Sciences*, 35, 512–520.

Ku, Y.-L., Kuo, S.-M., & Yao, C.-Y. (2010). Establishing the validity of a spiritual distress scale for cancer patients hospitalized in southern Taiwan. *International Journal of Palliative Nursing*, 16, 134–138.

Martins, H., & Caldeira, S. (2018). Spiritual distress in cancer patients: A synthesis of qualitative studies. *Religions*, 9, 285.

Monod, S., Martin, E., Spencer, B., Rochat, E., & Büla, C. (2012). Validation of the spiritual distress assessment tool in older hospitalized patients. *BMC Geriatrics*, 12, 1–9.

Monod, S. M., Rochat, E., Büla, C. J., Jobin, G., Martin, E., & Spencer, B. (2010). The spiritual distress assessment tool: An instrument to assess spiritual distress in hospitalised elderly persons. *BMC Geriatrics*, 10, 1–9.

Mrdjenovich, A. J. (2019). Religiously/spiritually involved, but in doubt or disbelief—Why? Healthy? *Journal of Religion and Health*, 58, 1488–1515.

Narayanasamy, A. (2006). The impact of empirical studies of spirituality and culture on nurse education. *Journal of Clinical Nursing*, 15, 840–851.

Pinho, C. M., Gomes, E. T., Trajano, M. d. F. C., Cavalcanti, A. T. d. A., Andrade, M. S., & Valença, M. P. (2017). Impaired religiosity and spiritual distress in people living with HIV/AIDS. *Revista Gaucha de Enfermagem*, 38, e67712.

Schultz, M., Meged-Book, T., Mashiach, T., & Bar-Sela, G. (2018). The cultural expression of spiritual distress in Israel. *Supportive Care in Cancer*, 26, 3187–3193.

Smucker, C. (1996). A phenomenological description of the experience of spiritual distress. *International Journal of Nursing Terminologies and Classifications*, 7, 81–91.

Simão, T. P., Chaves, E. C. L., & Iunes, D. H. (2015). Spiritual distress: The search for new evidence. *Revista de Pesquisa Cuidado é Fundamental Online*, 7, 2591–2602.

Sipon, S., Sakdan, M. F. a., Mustaffa, C. S., Marzuki, N. A., Khalid, M. S., Ariffin, M. T., Nazli, N. N. N. N., & Abdullah, S. (2015). Spirituality among flood victims: A comparison between two states. *Procedia-Social and Behavioral Sciences*, 185, 357–360.

Tanyi, R. A. (2002). Towards clarification of the meaning of spirituality. *Journal of Advanced Nursing*, 39, 500–509.

Velosa, T., Caldeira, S., & Capelas, M. L. (2017). Depression and spiritual distress in adult palliative patients: A cross-sectional study. *Religions*, 8, 156.

Yang, C. T., Narayanasamy, A., & Chang, S. L. (2012). Transcultural spirituality: The spiritual journey of hospitalized patients with schizophrenia in Taiwan. *Journal of Advanced Nursing*, 68, 358–367.

Author Biographies

The Rev. Dr. Lindsay Bates has been a member of the National Guild of Hypnotists since 1995 and is a past President of the Clergy Special Interest Group within the Guild. She is a member of the Order of Braid, an international honor society for the hypnotic arts and sciences. Hypnosis was a central tool in her pastoral ministry. Now retired after 40 years in the parish, she works in partnership with her spouse, the Rev. Dr. Charles Scot Giles, as the practice Reiki Master. She now blends hypnotic techniques with Reiki for her clients.

The Rev. Dr. C. Scot Giles is a senior member of the National Guild of Hypnotists. For more than thirty-five years he has maintained a large practice in hypnotic coaching that includes three free clinics for cancer patients in an arc around Chicago. He is the author of the curriculum used by the National Guild of Hypnotists to train colleagues to do hypnotic medical and cancer health coaching. He has won many awards, and in 2005 was inducted into the Order of James Braid, an international honor society for the hypnotic arts and sciences.

Celeste Hackett is an award winning professional Hypnotist, Life Coach and Hypnosis Instructor with a 24 year background as a major market radio personality. She is known for rapid success in working with people who have very difficult personal problems, her mastery of a complex hypnotic system called 5-PATH® and for building a thriving six figure hypnosis practice out of her home in Plano, Texas.

Rev. Timothy Jones worked in civil intelligence in Ontario, Canada for 28 years, trained in forensic hypnosis in 1986 and transitioned to clinical hypnotherapy in 2005. His life focus changed in 2000 with the death of his stepson, when he attended seminary. An NGH Certified Instructor, he teaches advanced and specialty courses to certified practitioners and with an active hypnotherapy practice in southern Ontario, Tim is considered an expert in the science with his focus on brief change work to quickly help modify behavior patterns no longer benefiting the client. With over two decades of clinical experience and a Baccalaureate and Masters in Christian Ministry, Tim is completing a PhD in Transpersonal Counseling with a focus on ameliorating the effects of attracted or randomly occurring energy attachments influencing human behavior within naturally occurring ego states.

Chris Lemig is a transpersonal hypnotherapist, author, and meditation teacher. Prior to pursuing a career in hypnotherapy, he spent several years as a Buddhist monk studying philosophy, meditation, and religious ritual in India and Nepal. He founded True Nature Hypnotherapy in 2019 where he works with private clients to heal past traumas and create powerful, healthy changes in their lives. In addition, he teaches a transformational workshop for emotional healing and spiritual growth called Gateway to the Limitless.

Rev. Christian Skoorsmith, MA, PsyD(c), FNGH, is an award-winning hypnotherapist and mental health professional in Seattle, Washington, USA. He is the author of five books on hypnosis and more than 50 articles in academic and professional journals. He is a popular speaker on hypnosis-related topics around the world, and was awarded the NGH Hypnotism Research Award for his pioneering work with tinnitus and the IAHP Science Award for scholarly rigor. Skoorsmith serves in leadership positions in the International Association of Hypnosis Professionals (IAHP) and the Clergy Special Interest Group of the NGH. He earned a Masters of Religion and served ten years in ministerial and executive leadership in Community of Christ, an international peace church, and is still ordained and active in congregational ministry. In 2016, he transitioned to hypnotherapy and in 2023 Skoorsmith was inducted as a Board Certified *Fellow* of the NGH – a distinction fewer than ¼ of 1% of hypnotists achieve. He maintains a successful hypnotherapy practice that The Seattle Times named "the best alternative therapy in the Pacific Northwest."

www.ingramcontent.com/pod-product-compliance
Lightning Source LLC
Chambersburg PA
CBHW060355290526
45791CB00002B/518